The Complete Guide to
TOTAL FITNESS

The Complete Guide to
TOTAL FITNESS

Jan Percival

Lloyd Percival

Joe Taylor

Methuen

New York   Toronto   London   Sydney

Published in the United States of America by Methuen, Inc., 572 Fifth Avenue, New York, N.Y. 10036, by arrangement with Prentice-Hall of Canada, Ltd.

Published simultaneously in Canada, by Prentice-Hall of Canada, Ltd., 1870 Birchmount Rd., Scarborough, Ontario M1P 2J7

Library of Congress Cataloging in Publication Data
Percival, Jan, 1947-
  The complete guide to total fitness.

  1. Exercise. 2. Physical fitness. I. Percival, Lloyd, joint author. II. Taylor, Joseph W., joint author. III. Title.
RA781.P47 1977   613.7   77-9867
ISBN 0-458-92980-8

DESIGN: William Fox/Associates
ILLUSTRATION: Helen Fox
PHOTOGRAPHY: Harold Whyte
PHOTO OF LLOYD PERCIVAL: Barry Stewart Associates
COMPOSITION: Webcom
Printed and bound in Canada by the John Deyell Company

Contents

FITNESS AND EXERCISE

FITNESS AND DAILY LIVING

FITNESS FOR CHILDREN

Acknowledgments

The authors are grateful for the assistance of editor Marta Tomins whose personal interest in fitness made her contribution invaluable. A special note of appreciation goes to models Nadja Cochrane, Joan Bain, Dave Watts, John Henderson, and our child wonders, Charlene Traviss and Chris Welch, for reminding us that fitness can be fun.

Preface

Lloyd Percival was fond of telling people: "Get fit, and you'll enjoy your vices more." It says a lot about the man; more, perhaps, than a recitation of his achievements and capabilities. His sense of mission never outweighed his sense of humanity; his message was not one to be preached dogmatically from a pulpit. Life was for living, and for living well. Sport was for fun and the pursuit of excellence. Human frailties were to be disregarded because human strength, dignity, and spirit outweighed them.

In the end, his own frailties triumphed far earlier than he deserved. The recognition for which he struggled long and hard came late. He was regarded by many as Canada's foremost coaching and fitness authority and yet he died at 61, still seeking new conquests, far too unwilling to relax and contemplate his achievements.

This book is based on his work in fitness. It is not exactly the book he had planned to write – much of that remained in his unique mind, a mind with an uncanny ability to synthesize scientific knowledge for the man on the street. But in his writings and his speeches, and in the minds of those who were associated with him, he left enough to produce what we fondly believe is a book he would have liked to have written.

What is the point of being fit, you may ask, if a man like Lloyd Percival can die in his early 60s? The point is this: It was through a fitness campaign many years ago that he regained his own health and despite medical problems, was able to prolong his life. This campaign put to the test many of his ideas on fitness and culminated in the founding of the world-famous Fitness Institute in Toronto.

He once wrote: "Most authorities who prepare programs on how to keep fit are perfect examples of what a regular fitness program can do. It is my opinion, however, that a person who has always been fit is perhaps not aware of the problems, attitudes, and circumstances influencing the unfit. He is too disdainful of their weaknesses; he is not sufficiently aware of the very real difficulties facing them.

"It is here that I feel I have a definite advantage. As far as condition, or the lack of it, is concerned I have run the gamut."

Lloyd Percival was a complex man. He was a coach, confidant, iconoclast, athlete, intellectual, wit, egotist, father figure, critic, innovator, and early Canadian nationalist. He was controversial, outspoken, and in and out of hot water with the establishment as often as he was in and out of the newspaper headlines. He died, as Jim Proudfoot of the Toronto Star wrote, "when all his old adversaries were ready for defeat. He died when Canada was at last ready for him." Typically, he was wearing many hats on that July day in 1974: he was planning a multimillion dollar national fitness campaign; providing training programs for many of Canada's top athletes and teams in a diversity of sports; acting as advisor to the Canadian Olympic Association; publishing his own monthly sports and fitness newspaper; planning books on fitness, coaching, and training for hockey – and promoting a pop group.

The people who knew Lloyd well called him "Coach". Even in his early days as an athlete he'd wanted, someday, to tell Canadians how to run, jump, and play properly. He'd played almost all of the major sports himself, some of them exceptionally well: he was Canada's leading cricketer, a golden gloves boxing champ, a finalist in the Canadian junior tennis championships, a good hockey, lacrosse, and football player, and a track and field athlete. He studied at the Sokol Institute in Prague, Loughborough College and Kings College in England, and the universities of Wisconsin and Southern California in the United States. His courses were varied: physiology, psychology, principles of coaching, principles of salesmanship (from legendary football coach Knute Rockne), physical education, sports medicine.

In 1941 he and his bride, Dorothy, passed up a honeymoon to buy time on radio for an enterprise he called "Sports College". It eventually became a coast-to-coast broadcast carried by the CBC network for nearly 21 years, the beginning and the basis of his lifelong campaign to educate Canadians on sports, fitness, and anything else he thought they should know about physical activity. He wrote hundreds of thousands of words which appeared in dozens of books, booklets, and pamphlets distributed through Sports College to millions of people over the years.

In 1946, Coach organized the Toronto Red Devils Track Club, and embarked on a career which earned him recognition as one of Canada's outstanding coaches. As usual, he was ahead of his time. John Hudson, executive director of the Coaching Association of Canada – an organization born of a 1969 Percival brief to the government – commented: "His runners were into interval training 15 years before anybody else here."

In 1950, Coach wrote his authoritative *Hockey Handbook*. Many hockey men of that day scoffed because they didn't understand it. But the Russians understood, and adapted it as the basis of their development program. The architect of Soviet hockey, Anatoli Tarasov, inscribed a copy of his own book to Coach, thanking him for "your wonderful book which introduced us to the mysteries of Canadian hockey . . . I have studied it like a schoolboy."

Coach launched his national "get fit" campaign in the early 50s, an era when Canadians were reluctant to hear warnings about the dangers of a lifetime of inactivity. Yet, when the $2.5 million Fitness Institute was inaugurated in 1969 it was, to quote one writer, "an idea whose time had come". With its array of scientific testing and measuring equipment, skilled staff, and Coach's expertise in devising training and conditioning programs, the Fitness Institute soon became a mecca not only for obese citizens seeking to regain their lost youth but also for athletes of all persuasions. Golfers George Knudson and Al Balding, Olympic divers Bev Boys and Nancy Robertson, skaters Karen Magnussen and Val and Sandra Bezic, the national ski team and countless others sought training advice or programs to rehabilitate damaged limbs and ligaments.

Honors which had eluded him for so long now began to accumulate. He was named a member of the International Society for Physical Education, the International Trainers Association, the International Federation of Sport and Fitness Medicine, the International Coaches Association, the American College of Sport Medicine and, posthumously, the Canadian Sports and Boxing Halls of Fame.

"Like Banting and Best, he was self-taught, and we must respect his single-mindedness of purpose and the devotion of his whole life to physical fitness", said Dr. Paul McGoey, one of Canada's outstanding surgeons.

Dr. Ernst Jokl, president of the Research Committee of the International Council of Sport and Physical Education, described him as the bridge between science and the ordinary citizen: "What you and your daughter and your helpers have demonstrated is that facilities can and must be placed at the disposal of Mr. and Mrs. Everybody", he wrote in 1972.

This book is dedicated to Lloyd Percival's memory in the hope that it can become a part of that bridge, a sort of "facility" which Mr. and Mrs. Everybody can take home and which may, perhaps, help them to feel younger, healthier, and more confident next year than they do right now. As Coach wrote in the introduction to one of his fitness publications:

"I know how you feel, fit or unfit. I think I understand your problems, especially if you are very busy and harassed by the thought that tomorrow will bring an even tougher load for a body you know to be weakening. I know that you can 'come back', that you can get fit and stay fit, that you *can* regain your confidence in your body.

"What you want is to be fit enough to do your job without undue fatigue and tension, to have enough energy for recreation and to know that you are doing something practical to postpone the process of aging. Actually, it isn't so tough!"

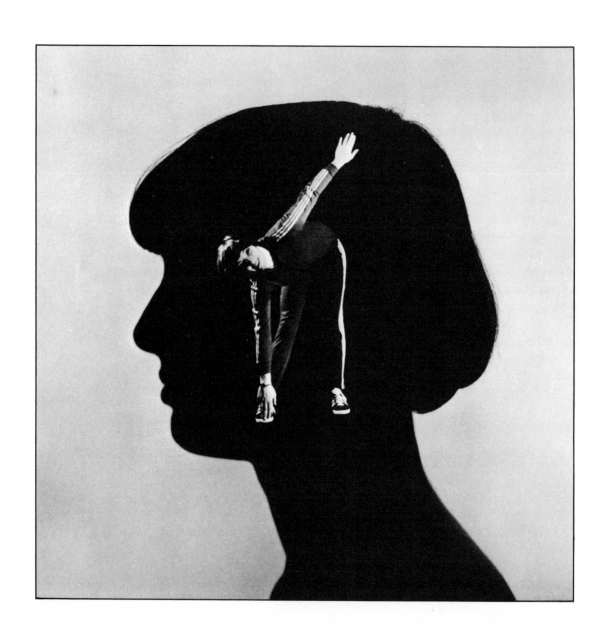

Fitness and You

1

It's Easy Once You Know How

WHAT IS FITNESS?

If you were to ask 20 people the meaning of physical fitness, you would get 20 different answers. Fitness is all things to all people, a precious commodity which enables us to live our lives to the full yet is really cherished only when it begins to fade away. To an older person, it might be the feeling of youthful vigor, to an athlete the capacity to run a mile in four minutes, to a stenographer the ability to type for eight hours at a stretch without developing aching shoulder muscles. To a coach it is something which comes with training, to a physician it is a functional state of the body defined in technical terms.

It is all these things, and more. It is strength, flexibility, agility, power, speed, and muscular and cardiovascular endurance. It is the ability to enjoy our daily lives and to achieve our goals without undue fatigue or stress. It is having a reserve of physical stamina and strength for safety and the enjoyment of leisure activities. It is protection against degenerative diseases, and feeling physically youthful even when we are growing old.

Fitness is active, not passive. Yet recent decades have seen a quantum leap in the number of devices which help us to avoid effort and movement, the two key ingredients in physical fitness. We can no longer take fitness for granted, as could people of an earlier era, because the automatic movements which should maintain it — walking, carrying, pushing, running, jumping, digging, lifting — are gradually becoming unnecessary. We don't even have to get to our feet to change television programs.

It's only human to take advantage of short cuts. But even though many of us are beginning to recognize the need to combat the rising toll of degenerative diseases and the decrease in capacity for activities which require effort, all too often we still look for a button to push. We want to get fit without having to work at it and without making changes in our life styles. This is not possible.

What must be done, then? The first step is to accept the need for fitness and to make a personal commitment. The second is to understand the degree of fitness required by our own particular life style, and the third is to find a program which suits our physical needs, time, and personality, and to follow it through.

Most of us tend to "compartmentalize" fitness. We think in terms of being able to run a mile in x number of minutes, or playing tennis better than Fred next door, or fitting into our clothes without bulging in embarrassing places, or just staying alive until next year. It's as if each function of our bodies were separate from the others.

But there is no way we can train one isolated physiological mechanism and still make ourselves *totally* fit. Some aspects of fitness are more important than others, but if we are to function at full efficiency we have to treat the body as a single entity which stands or falls on its weakest part, whether that part be the strength of the abdominal muscles, posture, heart-wind endurance, back-thigh flexibility, or eating habits.

This is why a fitness program which consists solely of jogging, cycling, swimming, or any other single activity is not totally effective. It may be better than nothing, but it will not be adequate in the overall context. What value is there in running a mile in seven minutes if back problems give you constant pain? What purpose is there in having the strength to lift 150 lbs. overhead if cardiovascular problems make it a health hazard to do so? What pleasure is there in fitting into a new outfit if you haven't the energy and endurance to go out and enjoy wearing it?

On the other hand, what's the point in acquiring physical fitness if the effort involved demands all your spare time and willpower?

Somewhere, there's a middle ground, an answer that's right for you – a way of acquiring all the important elements of fitness without pushing you to the limits of your character and determination. This book does not tell you that you can get fit in just three minutes a day, nor does it provide a taxing program which, if rigidly followed, will guarantee three inches off your waistline. But it does show you how you can develop your own program to meet your own needs in your own time and at your own pace – and stay with it.

Let's examine the values of fitness more closely.

What Level of Fitness Do You Need?

You need sufficient fitness for:

1. Functional ability to protect you now and in the future from those ailments which relate directly to functional inability. These include many heart problems, high blood pressure and other circulatory ailments, osteoporosis (bone deterioration), degenerative diseases in general, stomach and abdominal problems, low back pain, stress-induced diseases such as anxiety, ulcers and many emotional problems, and numerous other common afflictions that appear to be on the increase in our society. The general descriptive term for all these symptoms is "hypokinetic disease" – "hypo" meaning abnormally low or deficient, "kinetic" meaning of, or produced by motion; that is, disease produced by abnormally low levels of physical activity.

2. Safety. Not only is the fit person less likely to be involved in accidents, he or she is more likely to survive them without serious injury and to recover more quickly from aftereffects. Strength, endurance, reaction time, agility, and flexibility all help to protect against accident and injury. The phrase "survival of the fittest" is still valid.

3. A full life span. The objective link between fitness and longevity has not been proven to the satisfaction of the scientist. But there is strong evidence that fit people do live longer. We lose what we don't use. According to Dr. Laurence E. Morehouse: "Body structures and functions adjust to the load placed on them. When the load is diminished, muscles waste away and strength is lost. The heart becomes smaller, weaker, and less efficient. Blood vessels disappear. The storage of energy chemicals decreases. As a result, the body becomes less capable of meeting physical demands, and may fail in emergency situations."[1]

4. Enough energy to handle your daily work load without stress and discomfort and

a reserve of energy for hobbies, recreation, and those special emergencies which arise from time to time, both at work and at home.

5. Optimum earning power. Fit people can concentrate better, work longer, withstand pressure better, miss fewer work days, and create a better all-round impression on others. By keeping their ambition, drive, and vitality longer, fit people extend their peak working years. All this means potentially improved income.

6. A happy life style. When you are fit, you look better, feel better, and are likely to have more physical energy. When you feel fit, the good things of life have more meaning: the sky is bluer, the music sweeter, the steak tastier, and you can even enjoy your vices more. This is true because all parts of the body are operating at full efficiency. You can work or play harder, and recover faster.

7. A full domestic life. Most sociologists are aware that fit people are less irritable, less tense, and less easily upset. They have more energy to play with their children, share domestic duties, and be more responsive to their partners sexually and emotionally.

Are You As Fit As You Think You Are?

There is evidence that the average urban-dweller in an industrialized society is not as fit as he or she should be to enjoy a healthy, active life free from diseases caused by degeneration of body tissues. If you are 35 years old, you are likely to be middle-aged from a physiological viewpoint. Age should be measured by the responses of the body rather than by the passing of years. Men and women will deteriorate physically between the ages of 25 and 35 more than in any other decade of their lives.

Here are some of the results of measurements and tests conducted at a fitness center in Toronto.

The two most important physiological changes measured were a 50 per cent increase in the fat content of the body and a 27 per cent decrease in the maximum oxygen uptake. The latter is the body's ability to take in and utilize oxygen during physical effort and is generally considered to be the single most significant component of fitness.

Also noted were the following:

Heart performance: 24 per cent decrease

Posture (observable problems): 27 per cent increase

Flexibility: 21 per cent decrease

Strength: 14 per cent decrease

Those who had been sedentary during this dangerous decade showed definite tendencies toward the high risk factors which so intrigue insurance companies: elevated blood pressure, increased blood (serum) cholesterol and triglyceride levels, emotional instability (anxieties), and obesity.

The message is clear. If you are in the dangerous decade, or if you passed through it with a minimum of physical activity, you probably should start evaluating your fitness level in terms of an emergency. As you get older, the body loses its ability to tolerate degenerative stresses and begins to break down. The time to start doing something about it is now. If you do not, you are laying down a pattern of physiological deterioration which might very well mean that your future years will be neither as healthy, productive, nor enjoyable as they should be.

YOUR FITNESS PRIORITIES

You can lose an arm or a leg and still function fairly efficiently; you can even become extremely fit. The sports world contains a surprising number of athletes who have triumphed over severe disabilities. But you cannot lose your heart and stay alive, nor your strength and remain upright. You cannot be totally fit if one of the *essential* components of the body is not functioning efficiently. Consequently, there are certain fitness priorities:

- cardiorespiratory fitness
- nutrition
- abdominal fitness
- strength
- relaxation
- flexibility
- motor efficiency

Cardiorespiratory Fitness

The heart is a pump, while the arteries and veins are fuel lines which feed life-giving fluids to the working muscles, organs, and brain. The heart, lungs, and circulation are inextricably linked together — the three musketeers of physical well-being. "One for all and all for one" sums up their relationship perfectly. A fitness campaign which neglects any one of these components is not really a fitness campaign at all.

Just as any fitness campaign should begin with a medical checkup in which tests of heart fitness play an important part, so a *scientifically* planned fitness program should begin with an oxygen-uptake test which measures the efficiency with which the lungs extract oxygen from the air and the circulation distributes it throughout the body. Oxygen is the body's fuel.

Sedentary living seriously decreases the capacity to utilize oxygen, throwing a terrific strain on the heart, which must work harder and harder as the years go by in order to supply all the vital organs: the muscles, the stomach, the brain, the kidneys, liver, glands. Sometimes even the slightest exertion can throw a dangerous load on the heart, particularly if the arteries are clogged with cholesterol compounds and there are miles and miles of surplus blood vessels contained in excess fatty tissues.

In the extremes of this situation the heart is even unable to pump enough blood to supply itself adequately (after all, the heart is a muscle) and a heart attack results.

There have been attempts to prove that physical activity does not prevent coronary heart disease; some authorities argue that your physical and emotional patterns predispose you to cardiac risk even if you do get sufficient exercise.

This may be true. Even heart-attack victims who have become so fit (training under medical supervision, by the way — don't try it on your own) that they can compete in marathon runs are not immune to further cardiac accidents. But — and this is an important point — they are more likely to survive such attacks, and to recover more quickly, and live a more normal life afterwards than those who are physically unfit.

There is strong evidence that exercise, particularly a moderate level of exercise throughout life, can help to reduce the incidence of heart disease. Exercise is particularly useful in reducing the manifestations of atherosclerosis (fatty build up in the vessels) and arteriosclerosis (hardening), two major causes of heart attacks and strokes.

After an extensive study of heart disease, Doctors Samuel M. Fox and John L. Byer of the Research Committee of the President's Council on Physical Fitness and Sports supported the value of physical activity in reducing the incidence and severity of and mortality from chronic heart disease.

The effects of regular vigorous exercise on the heart and circulatory system include the following:

1. An increase in the number of capillaries as well as the use of latent capillaries, resulting in improved endurance.

2. A decrease in resting heart rate and an increase in stroke volume. The heart thus has more chance to rest while pumping the required amount of blood throughout the body.

3. A shortening of the heart's recovery time following exercise. This indicates that the

body is able to adjust more quickly to physical stress.

4. An increase in cardiac output, blood volume, and red-cell count, allowing more oxygen to reach the muscles. This results in greater work performance.

5. Increases in the amount of oxygen picked up by the blood in the lungs owing to increased capillarization, and consequent increases in supplies to the muscles.

6. More efficient removal of lactic acid from the tissues, thereby delaying and reducing fatigue, and aiding recovery from effort.

7. Reduction of blood cholesterol formation and a decrease in fatty lipids in the blood, reducing the potential for the development of atherosclerosis.

8. Decreased blood pressure.

9. Increased elasticity of artery walls.

Although heart disease may have many causes, lack of regular exercise seems to be a major culprit. Exercise of the right kind and of the right frequency is good preventive medicine, and helps to neutralize such contributory risk factors as smoking, obesity, and tension. However, spasmodic exercise such as weekend tennis or skiing, does not provide this preventive factor and can be stressful if it is fairly strenuous.

Nutrition

Nutrition is in many respects the single most important factor in fitness. Your eating habits are one of the first things your doctor will regulate if you are prey to such ailments as elevated cholesterol levels, high blood pressure and other cardiovascular diseases, ulcers, obesity, anemia, some eye problems, and certain nervous and emotional difficulties. Twenty per cent of the participants in a $2.5 million Nutrition Canada study had to be referred to doctors for treatment of symptoms related to nutritional deficiencies—a staggering number in an affluent society.

Survey after survey has shown that the nutritional pattern of the average person living in a modern technological society, particularly the young person, is badly out of balance. Millions of people are literally ''eating themselves sick''. Malnutrition can exist long before the symptoms show. Persistant colds, low energy and stamina, high anxiety levels and lack of resistance to infections may be warning signs.

We are deluged with literature on nutrition, ranging from long treatises on the effects of Vitamin C on intelligence to the uses of alfalfa sprouts and kelp. In between, there is the ''balanced diet'' – although many people who think they're on one probably are not – which simply requires sensible eating habits and an awareness of what calories, vitamins, minerals and other elements we need and where to get them in adequate quantities. Eat according to your needs and avoid too much of certain foods high in elements which have been found to be inimical to health and fitness, such as cholesterol and refined sugar.

In certain cases, some supplementation of vitamins and minerals may be required as well, and you should know about the need for replenishment after strenuous activity. It is not the intention of this book to delve into the more esoteric areas of diet, or into highly contentious issues such as the megavitamin theory. Chapter 7, Nutrition, is designed to provide a sound, sensible guide to general nutrition for maximum health and fitness, as well as weight control.

Posture

The prevalence of low back pain and other orthopedic abnormalities makes us realize the importance of good posture to our continued health and well-being.

Good or bad posture usually stems from habits developed while young. Careless attitudes in sitting and standing become magnified as the years pass and the body becomes increasingly incapable of withstanding the steady downward drag of gravity. Many of the chronic diseases of the middle-aged and the elderly can be traced directly to posture. These are the "fifth column disorders that sneak up on us as silent saboteurs"[2] says Dr. Edward Stieglitz.

According to the *Encyclopedia of Sport Sciences and Medicine*: "Most disease in later years is insidious in onset and slow but persistent in progression. Circulatory and vascular diseases lead the list, which also includes metabolic and joint diseases. All are exaggerated by bad posture. Even some mental disorders are increased by interference with good circulation of blood to the brain."[3]

It is apparent, then, that continued good health is one very important reason for maintaining correct posture. There is another, equally important reason: appearance and self-image.

Dr. Katharine F. Wells points out in *Posture Exercise Handbook* that good posture influences the attitude you have toward yourself. It also "inspires the confidence of others because it reflects the degree of your own self-confidence and self-respect".[4]

Dr. Wells lists the following as the most important elements of good posture when you are standing erect:

1. Total body weight is centered squarely above both feet or else is very slightly forward, but never backward.

2. Major weight-bearing segments of the body (the lower extremities, pelvis, trunk) and the head are aligned either vertically or slanting very slightly forward.

3. Pelvis is centered squarely above the feet and beneath the trunk, providing firm support for the latter.

4. Chest is slightly lifted but the elevation is not forced.

5. Head is erect with the profile vertical and the chin level.

6. Feet point forward or slightly outward. In walking they point straight ahead.

7. Ankles, as seen from the front or back, are straight. There is neither pronation (inward sagging) nor supination (exaggerated cupping or arching).

8. Total posture is maintained without evidence of strain or tension.

Even people who have had good posture all their lives find it increasingly difficult to maintain if they allow their muscles to lose strength and tone. The body depends on the holding forces of muscles and ligaments to remain in alignment; when these forces diminish, gravity starts to win the battle.

Prolonged poor posture makes it impossible to regain a proper, erect position without training. Certain muscles need to be returned to a state of strength and flexibility in order to do their job without fatigue. Others, which may have shortened, need to be stretched before they will allow the bones to return to their proper places. This is why lack of flexibility in the back thigh muscles (common among people who sit all day) and in the muscles of the chest (common if you hunch over a desk) are among the hazards to continued good health.

Many of the exercises in this book, particularly those contained in Chapter 6, 'Special Problems', relate specifically to posture problems. An active life style in which walking, swimming, sports, and other physical activities are prominent also plays a central role in maintaining good posture, increasingly so as the years pass by.

Parents should pay particular attention to their children's posture. In this area more than almost any other, an ounce of prevention is worth years of cure.

Abdominal Fitness

One of the first parts of the body to provide visible evidence of physical degeneration is the stomach, both above and below the belt. Your midsection should be one of the primary targets of your fitness campaign. There are several reasons:

1. It is a favorite dumping area for excess fat. Everyone accumulates fat in slightly different ways which are a result of inherited body type and accustomed patterns of activity. The stomach is a particularly noticeable site.

2. The muscles of the stomach carry a heavy load and are at constant war with the forces of gravity as they struggle to hold the stomach and other organs in position. Eventually, if posture habits are poor and muscle tone disappears, everything starts to sag. This "abdominal prolapse" can lead to many complications, with digestive problems ranking high among them. Low back pain is another common result because the proper alignment of the back depends on the holding power of the sinews which keep the pelvis where it belongs, and abdominal muscles are chief among them.

Too much fat in the abdominal area forces posture changes as the body struggles to compensate for extra weight up front. The curve of the lower back is increased, squeezing the vertebrae and putting extra pressure on the discs and nerves in this area. Other compensating posture defects develop (an equal and opposite curve in the upper back, for example).

Strength

Strength is one of the forgotten fitness fundamentals. People tend to think that strength is useful for putting the shot or pinning an opponent to the mat; "but", they conclude, "what do *I* need to build muscles for? All I do is sit in a chair all day."

The loss of strength has many ramifications:

- 85 per cent of all back problems are traceable directly to lack of muscular strength, particularly in the abdominal muscles.

- Neuromuscular coordination diminishes; physical work of any kind demands extra effort.

- Muscular endurance is reduced; you tire more quickly.

- Joints lose stability, resulting in increased susceptibility to injury.

- Muscular sag increases and it becomes progressively more difficult to sustain proper posture; this, in turn, affects many of the internal organs as well as throwing stress on the back and other parts of our framework.

- The reserve of strength with which we handle physical emergencies is dissipated; our sense of physical security diminishes and we start to feel "old". Self-image suffers, and morale decreases.

- Body contours change. Even for women, proper muscular development produces and sustains a pleasing, youthful physical appearance. Loss of muscular development and tone causes us to look old before our time.

The average, untrained person reaches peak strength levels in his or her late teens or early 20s. Thereafter strength gradually decreases unless regular physical activity is sustained. Fortunately, muscular strength can be regained even at an advanced age. An organized, progressive program will do the job quite quickly. Once attained, strength is easily sustained with far less effort than was necessary to acquire it.

There's no need to build big muscles, either. Dr. Herbert deVries of California[5] likens the muscles, which are composed of numbers of fibers, to a team of dogs harnessed to a sled. To make the team more powerful you can either get bigger dogs (build the size of the individual fibers), or harness more dogs (increase the activation levels of the nervous system). We cannot augment the number of fibers since this is fixed at birth, but we can increase the *activation* of existing fibers when more strength is required, and we can also develop the skill with which they are activated.

For the average person then, strength gains depend upon improved neuromuscular activation which is best achieved by exercise that involves a relatively high number of repetitions at good speed without too much resistance. This not only produces strength but muscle endurance as well and helps to reduce fatty tissues. For those seeking bulk, the opposite principle holds true: fewer repetitions and greater resistance.

There are many ways to increase strength which are discussed in more detail in later chapters.

Relaxation

Tension, anxiety, and other manifestations of stress are symptomatic of the high-pressure, low-activity life style most of us lead. Before sitting down became a way of life, people had a physical outlet for many of society's pressures. Now we have nervous breakdowns.

Stress can age you prematurely. Stress can kill you. Conversely, a complete lack of stress can kill you too. The body and mind require a certain degree of tension to stay fit and healthy. We cannot simply vegetate.

Dr. Hans Selye describes physiological stress as "the non-specific response of the body to any demand made on it".[6] The body reacts to stress in three stages. First, when a demand is made – a request from the boss for an important report, for example – there is an initial "alarm" reaction. There are changes in blood concentration, an inflammatory response by certain internal organs, tensing of the muscles and so on. The second stage is one of adaptation and resistance – as you start to work on the report, the body begins to function more normally. The third stage – the dangerous one – is the exhaustion stage.

This is reached if the stress is not resolved after a period of time. Suppose, for example, that you are unable to produce an adequate report and your whole career may be in jeopardy. When this situation is prolonged or repeated you may experience ulcers, headaches, and possibly cardiovascular problems.

Muscular tension, then, is only one response to stress. In *affective* tension the tensing of the muscles is unconscious, possibly the result of anxiety, as in the attempt to meet a deadline. Coordination tension is caused by poor muscular coordination (this usually occurs in skilled activities which have not been well-learned). The type of tension most people are concerned with is affective tension.

What does tension do to you? Try this experiment: clench your fist hard. Watch how the knuckles turn white. Pressure on the blood vessels has squeezed blood away from certain areas. When your muscles are tense, they are producing the same effect in many parts of the body. If, for example, your neck and shoulder muscles are tense while you are typing a report, the circulation to the brain may be restricted. Tension in the stomach area may affect digestion. A general state of tension in the body may send blood pressure up. You find it hard to sleep, yet you are tired all the time simply because the muscles are continually at work – they never get a chance to relax and rest. Chronically tense people even have tight muscles when they sleep – they grind their teeth, clench their hands, and awake feeling fatigued. No wonder!

Relaxation is one answer – the art of getting rid of accumulated tension and of operating calmly in stressful or emotional situations without developing an excessive muscular response. Fortunately, it is an art which can be learned.

Regular exercise is another answer. During exercise the body finds an outlet for its tensions; it quickly reaches the adaptation and resistance stage. While exercise itself is a stress, done regularly and progressively, it is a beneficial one which teaches the body to resist stress and to adapt to it so that it never moves on to the exhaustion stage. When the body learns to handle the types of stress imposed by exercise, it quickly adapts to the non-specific stresses that are produced by sudden, abnormal conditions. According to Dr. Selye, there is a direct link between a person's physical fitness and his ability to adapt to business pressures, social stress, and emotional overloads as well as to his ability to recuperate more quickly from injury or disease.

Flexibility

The skeleton is held together by ligaments — tough bands of tissue which circle the joints and keep the bones in place — and by muscles which are attached to the bones by tendons. When these lose their functional efficiency, and when muscles become shortened and tense, we not only look older, we *feel* older. It takes longer to get going in the morning; we feel stiff and creaky during and after exercise; it gets harder to perform certain movements such as putting on shoes and stockings, and it seems more difficult to stand up straight. The old spring and bounce is gone — but not forgotten, nor irretrievably lost. Muscles and tendons which have become tense and inflexible through lack of use can quite quickly and easily be put right. This is why stretching exercises for the major muscles of the body are an essential part of any good fitness program. Particularly important are the back thigh muscles, the muscles of the lower back, and the large muscles of the chest and rib cage.

The joints must also be exercised through their full range — backward, forward, and around in a rotating action when this is the joint's natural pattern of movement.

Motor Efficiency

Our neuromuscular efficiency governs the skill with which we are able to use our bodies. Learned patterns of behavior range from the very basic movements such as walking, grasping objects, and eating with a knife and fork to the highly complex skills of the trained athlete, the musician, and the ballet dancer. We all need some degree of neuromuscular coordination to function efficiently and without fatigue; moreover, there is strong evidence that general motor ability degenerates through disuse. Loss of physical skills is also a symptom of the aging process. We feel old because we perform as if we were old. A physically active life style is important for all of us.

Physical activity is even more important for the young child. Motor skills must be learned. The child who is inactive, who watches television at the expense of more active play, and who seldom participates in the rough-and-tumble of the formative years, not only fails to develop basic motor skills, he or she also fails to develop adequate physical equipment (muscles, neurological patterns) with which to perform these skills later on. Because there is a link between motor and mental ability, children with learning disabilities are now given special physical training programs.

These, then, are your priority targets. If the requirements sound a bit complex, take heart because they are not. All exercise affects one or more of these priorities; some exercises condition and develop all of them. The efficient organization of activity to match your specific, individual needs will be explained in this book. What is essential for you at this stage is *awareness*: awareness of the need for regular physical activity, and awareness of what it can do for you.

2

Keeping
Your Body Young

The nature of life demands that our bodies grow old, but most of us feel and act old before our time. We lose or waste precious years of youth. Five out of six North Americans are older physiologically than they are chronologically. What's the point of celebrating a 30th birthday, for example, if our muscles and heart and lungs say we're 40?

It's bad enough that certain degenerative diseases can flourish when we let the physical machinery run down. The greatest loss of all is that feeling of youthfulness — of free and easy movement and of limitless energy. ''You're as old as you feel'' is a saying that makes sound, physiological sense.

Chronological time cannot be turned back. Physiological time can. It's possible to be physically younger one year from now than you are today. The answer lies in sound nutrition, a relaxed attitude to life, and regular muscular activity for the key factors which keep you feeling young: flexibility, heart-wind efficiency, circulation, posture, motor ability, and strength.

WHAT EXERCISE CAN DO FOR YOUR BODY

The body's adaptive mechanism is a wonder. Most people do not understand precisely how efficient it is, and what it can do if given the chance. Dr. P. V. Karpovich conducted an experiment at Springfield College in which a group of men was given training on a bicycle ergometer. This is a stationary bicycle with attachments which allow the amount of work done to be measured accurately. In 22 weeks, working out 5 times a week, some men were able to improve their work output by as much as 4,400 per cent.

Think of what this means in terms of physical efficiency, of improved function in all the muscles, of the heart, the circulation and so on! But also think what this means in terms of inactivity. The body is capable of adapting to idleness just as fast as it adapts to activity. In 22 weeks those same men could lose 4,400 per cent of their work capability just by doing nothing. Far too many of us are in this category.

Dr. Bengt Saltin of Sweden carried out studies in which he found that individuals who remained in bed for as little as 3 weeks suffered 20 to 30 per cent decreases in maximum oxygen uptake (VO_2 max — the ability of the body to take in and utilize oxygen).

Other studies of prolonged bed rest have shown drastic, but fortunately reversible, effects on physiological functions, including loss of calcium from the bones and a decrease in muscle strength and bulk.

Dr. Laurence Morehouse points out that after 3 weeks in bed our fitness level becomes so low that there is a training effect from the first few steps we take when we get up.

VO$_2$ max is just one aspect of fitness, albeit an important one. The body adapts to regular exercise in other ways. In addition to improvements in the priority areas we discussed earlier, there will be changes in strength and muscle endurance, metabolism, cholesterol levels, blood pressure, and many of the various physiological functions which we regard as characteristic of youthfulness.

One of the primary concerns of the sedentary person should be the effect of inactivity upon his or her muscles. Muscles atrophy at an alarming rate when they're not used. As an extreme example, when a limb is immobilized in a cast, atrophy can begin within 24 hours. The muscles can decrease in size by half within a month. It is not even necessary to wear a cast. A person with a knee injury which causes him to favor the leg may find after a few weeks that the circumference of that thigh is an inch or two smaller.

The effect on the heart is the same. An athlete in good training may lose up to 200 cubic centimetres (12 cubic inches) of heart volume if forced to remain in bed for a few weeks. Similarly, an active person who becomes sedentary loses heart volume, and a person who is sedentary all his life simply never develops his heart to its full potential.

Anyone who has built up muscles through weight training (this bulking up of muscles is called hypertrophy) will lose most of that bulk after he stops specific strength work. Women training for such events as the shot put need not worry about too much bulk; most of it will disappear when training ends.

When training ends – for most people that period comes in their 20s when they become involved in a sedentary job and the problems of family life – this is when the aging process really begins. Fitness declines more between the ages of 25 and 35 than in any other decade, and atrophy, the chief weapon of the aging process, is the major cause. As we stop using our bodies, not only the muscles but the blood vessels, which carry oxygen, start to waste away.

No matter how big and strong they grow, muscles will not work for long without oxygen. This is why the efficiency of the heart and of the oxygen transport system are so important, and why maximum oxygen uptake is a key measure of fitness. The heart itself is a muscle; if it is deprived of oxygen for too long, it or parts of it cease to function.

The air we breathe is about 21 per cent oxygen. The efficiency of our lungs determines how much oxygen we extract from each breath. Lung size alone is not an accurate measure of our potential fitness. It is efficiency that counts.

As the oxygen enters the bloodstream at the lungs it combines with hemoglobin and is pumped by the heart to the muscles via the arteries. If we are anemic, there is less hemoglobin and thus less oxygen will enter the bloodstream.

The average person requires only three or four millilitres of oxygen per minute per kilogram of bodyweight while sitting in a chair. But once activity starts, the oxygen demand increases dramatically. In hard activity it may rise as much as 20 times.

That is why we get out of breath when we jog. The heart responds by pumping faster and we breathe more deeply and frequently. If we are not moving too fast, there is enough oxygen for the muscles to continue working and we can keep moving. The muscles "burn" carbohydrates and fat to release energy for contraction – the so-called "aerobic" (with air) process of metabolism – at the same rate as we supply oxygen. Theoretically we could keep going almost indefinitely at this "survival rate" if other factors were not involved.

Suppose we move faster and harder than our survival rate. The heart and the lungs are no longer capable of meeting the demands of the muscles for oxygen. The muscles keep going by utilizing certain fuel stores within the body, the most important being glycogen which is broken down after activity begins to supplement the energy supply. Lactic acid is produced. Eventually, the glycogen is used up, more and more lactic acid is produced, and fatigue sets in. The muscles fail to contract properly and coordination breaks down. (Fortunately, the healthy heart is able to keep going longer than the rest of our muscles.) This is the so-called "anaerobic" metabolic process – muscles functioning without sufficient oxygen. Competitive athletes know the feeling well. The sprint at the end of a close race pushes them near the limit at which complete muscle impairment takes place.

The circulatory system works hard to replace energy fuels and to clear lactic acid from the muscles, but if activity stops too soon there will be a residue left to irritate the nervous system. We feel stiff and sore for a day or two after unusual physical effort. Some lactic acid is still lurking about, and the nerve endings are objecting. A cooling-down period at the end of a training session helps the system to clear away the residues of effort by keeping the circulation moving at a slightly faster rate for a longer period of time. It also helps to replenish the used-up fuel supply.

The average unfit person goes into an anaerobic state much more quickly than one who has remained active; furthermore, the muscles have less tolerance for the situation when it does occur, and do not recover as fast. People who have not exercised for a long time are frequently shocked to find how much of their youthful endurance they have lost and react by avoiding further exertion. The *right* reaction is to start to work to regain endurance gradually with progressive exercise. Exercise doesn't have to hurt; when you find the method that's right for you, it becomes one of life's great pleasures.

Apart from training, one of the limiting factors to what we can do with our muscles is the composition of the muscles themselves. Research shows that, in general, we retain the numbers and types of muscle fibers that we had at birth. This is our genetic endowment. But remember the parable of the talents – what we do with those fibers is up to us. We can make them grow, or we can let them waste away.

Each of us has a certain number of red muscle fibers, and a certain number of white. It has been found that the red fibers move more slowly than the white but can keep moving longer, probably because they are better supplied with oxygen. White fibers are fast twitch fibers. If we have a high preponderance of them, we can become sprinters or athletes in other sports demanding speed. If we have a high proportion of red fibers, we may become long-distance runners. With a combination of both, we may be middle-distance runners or all-round athletes. However, speed tends to be specific to certain limbs—a fast runner is not necessarily able to throw fast, and vice versa.

The degree to which the fibers can be made to grow also seems to vary from individual to individual. Certain people can never bulk up like a heavyweight lifter no matter how hard they train, although they *can* become very strong. Neuromuscular activity plays a part here. The force of a muscular contraction is controlled by both the number and size of the fibers, and by the *moto-neurons* (motor nerve cells) which innervate or stimulate the fibers to contract. The force generated is affected by three factors other than size of fiber: 1. number of motor units (the moto-neuron and the fiber it innervates) recruited to exert the force, 2. rate of "firing" of the motor units, 3. synchronization or coordination of this firing. Training increases these three factors, and so the trained person with smaller muscles may use them more efficiently than an untrained bigger person. The biggest muscle is not necessarily the strongest.

Apart from the number and types of muscle fibers we have, the way in which we use them affects strength, endurance, speed, and skill of movement. Most of our muscles work in pairs. When one contracts, the other stretches. For example, when you lift something by bending your forearm at the elbow, the biceps contract to pull against the bones. At the same time, the triceps muscle on the bottom of the upper arm should relax to allow the arm to bend. In this case, the biceps is called the "agonist" muscle, while the triceps is the "antagonist"

When we lack skill in a movement, there is usually a certain amount of contraction in both the agonist and antagonist muscles. You can readily see how this affects skill – the muscles are working against each other. Endurance and speed are reduced since too many muscles are doing too much work, and strength is decreased. A person who trains to lift weights will usually be able to lift more weight than a person who may appear to be much bigger and stronger – he has learned to inhibit the action of the antagonist muscles which would otherwise "fight" against the movement. He has increased his skill of movement, which is one of the objectives of all training and practice, whether it be a small child learning to walk or an adult developing a new sports skill.

In general, women are genetically endowed with less strength than men – about one third less, according to research. Of course with training a woman can become as strong or stronger than a man who is sedentary.

According to Swedish physiologist Dr. Per-Olof Astrand,[1] maximal strength is attained between the ages of 20 and 30. After that there is a gradual decline to approximately 80 per cent of maximum at age 65. However, he says, habitual exercise and strength training will greatly retard this drop. If maximal strength has not been achieved in a person's 20s, he or she can become even stronger at age 65 than they were when younger by undertaking a strength development program.

Exercise and Blood Pressure

Blood pressure is expressed by two numbers, as follows: 120/80. The first figure represents the "systolic" pressure – the pressure of the blood against the walls of the arteries and veins when the heart is contracting and pumping out blood. The actual figure is the number of millimetres a column of mercury is forced up a pressure-measuring device.

The second figure is the "diastolic" pressure – the minimum pressure constantly present in the arteries even while the heart is resting between beats. It is generally considered to be the more significant of the two figures, since it represents a constant minimum.

What constitutes high blood pressure? This is something for your doctor to decide, since there are so many variables. Some people reach old age with blood-pressure levels which are extremely high when considered against the norm. Others have heart attacks or strokes despite only slight elevations in BP. The reasons are not fully understood. Bear this in mind, however: an estimated 10 per cent of North Americans have blood-pressure levels which are considered to be in the high risk area – and half of them are unaware of it. Make sure you have regular checkups, particularly if you are contemplating a fitness campaign.

There are four hollow chambers in the heart – two atria at the top and two ventricles at the bottom. When the heart "relaxes", blood enters the right atrium from the body, and the left atrium from the lungs. The atria then contract, squeezing the blood into the ventricles which then also contract, one sending blood through the main artery to the body, the other through the pulmonary artery to the lungs. Valves which slap shut at the proper moment keep the blood from backing up and make the sound you hear when you listen to your heart beat.

Under pressure, the blood will surge through the major arteries at up to 40 miles an hour; but it may take an entire minute to travel an inch in a capillary, while distributing food, chemicals, and oxygen into the body cells, and carrying away carbon dioxide and other waste products.

The body contains some 70,000 miles of arteries and tiny capillaries. Small blood vessels called arterioles expand or contract to control the flow of blood, much like the nozzle on a hose. (When you shut down the nozzle, you get less water but the pressure in the hose is higher.) Part of the process is normal; when you are running, for example, proportionately more blood flows to the legs and less to the stomach and brain because some arterioles open up and others close down. But if the arterioles are constantly shut down, blood pressure goes up and stays up. This is one of the initial causes of high blood pressure, and the exact reasons for it are still the subject of extensive research.

The name for high blood pressure is *hypertension* – high (hyper) pressure (tension) within the arteries.

Other factors involved in blood pressure are the output of the heart (cardiac output) and the kidneys. About one quarter of the heart's total output goes to the kidneys, and if there is a problem with circulation there, resistance to blood flow is increased and pressure goes up.

Two diseases usually associated with high blood pressure are: atherosclerosis (clogging of the arteries by fatty deposits) and arteriosclerosis (hardening of the arteries). While it is possible to have high blood pressure without the presence of either of these, their development will be accelerated and will in turn further increase the blood

pressure, leading to strokes and heart attacks. As the blood pressure increases and as the artery walls weaken and lose their elasticity, they are more likely to hemorrhage. Sometimes a portion will blow up like a small balloon, waiting for a small increase in pressure to cause it to burst. This is called an *aneurysm*.

The targets of high blood pressure, in addition to the blood vessels themselves, are organs such as the heart, kidneys, and brain. The eyes may also be affected, as well as the liver, kidneys, spleen, lungs, and adrenal glands.

Blood pressure increases during strenuous exercise because there is an increase in "cardiac output", the amount of blood the heart pumps. Cardiac output is the product of two things: heart rate (the speed at which it beats) and stroke volume (the amount of blood ejected with each beat). During exercise there is an increase in the size of blood vessels which helps reduce resistance to blood flow so that blood pressure does not shoot up as high as it otherwise might – unless your arteries are clogged with fatty byproducts and have lost their elasticity.

Arm work causes significantly higher blood

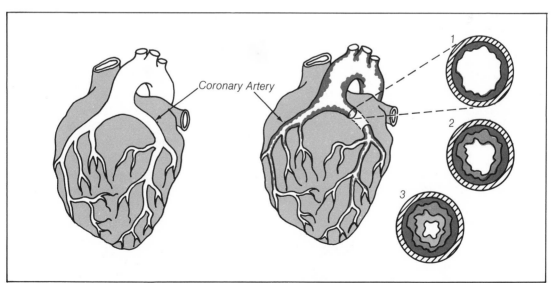

The Healthy Heart

The Atherosclerotic Heart
Three stages of coronary artery blockage are shown.

pressure than does leg work. When you are using your legs vigorously, the "milking" action of these big muscles aids the return of blood to the heart (venous return); this assistance is not so readily available during arm work and the heart must pump harder to compensate. Consequently, unfit persons or those suffering from cardiac ailments must be careful when they are shovelling snow, carrying heavy objects, or hammering nails overhead. They should also avoid weightlifting and isometric exercises because tensing of the muscles is often accompanied by a vaso-constriction which blocks blood flow.

The "Valsalva effect", named after an 18th-century Italian scientist, is another phenomenon associated with intense effort which can be dangerous for persons with heart problems. If you hold your breath during effort, the glottis (the space between the vocal chords at the upper part of the larynx) closes. This causes the pressure in the chest cavity to increase, preventing blood from returning to the heart. The heart, in effect, becomes starved for blood if the exertion continues for too long; blood pressure falls very quickly and the veins of the neck and head become distended. When exertion ends, the pressure shoots up to higher-than-normal levels.

Older persons and persons with heart-circulatory problems should be careful to breathe properly during exercise and other strenuous effort. Breath-holding exertions are out unless you know you are extremely fit, and the sudden rise and fall in blood pressure caused by the Valsalva effect will not lead to complications.

According to most of the textbooks, both systolic and diastolic blood pressures normally increase with age. But when two world-famous physiologists, Dr. Per-Olof Astrand of Sweden and Dr. Bruno Balke of the United States, undertook a long-term study of individuals who had kept fit, they found that there usually was no change in BP up to the age of 40, and in some cases up to age 70.

Why is this? There appear to be several reasons. First, regular exercise helps to open up blood vessels and also increases their number, thus decreasing resistance to blood flow. Not only does this help to keep blood pressure down during effort, but it promotes a faster return to normal afterwards. Exercise increases the size and elasticity of the large arteries. It also decreases resting heart rate and increases stroke volume, thus lightening the load on the heart.

Exercise helps to relieve tension and increase resistance to stress. Since anxiety and tension tend to elevate blood pressure, exercise provides a safety valve.

Exercise of the right type and duration can appreciably lower serum cholesterol levels. Vigorous leg and abdominal work has been found to produce the most favorable results. Isometric exercises, weightlifting, push-ups, and chinning the bar seem to have little effect, although they are valuable in other areas of fitness. Studies summarized in the *Physical Fitness Research Digest* (July 1974) indicated that at least 45 minutes of continuous cardiorespiratory endurance exercise was required. Five-times-a-week training produced better results than four, and four times was more efficient than three.

To have a marked effect on serum cholesterol levels, physical activity must be vigorous, continued for at least 45 minutes, and regular. Best results are obtained when nutrition is modified to decrease the intake of animal fats and increase consumption of vegetable oils (unsaturated fats).

According to Dr. Frank Finnerty Jr. and Shirley Motter Linde, high blood pressure is one reason a cholesterol-rich diet can be dangerous: "Animals fed a diet heavy with cholesterol will not have atherosclerosis if they have normal blood pressure. With high blood pressure that same diet — or even one lower in cholesterol — caused severe atherosclerosis in the animals and often led to heart attacks. A high cholesterol diet had an adverse effect *only* if the animal had high blood pressure."[2]

Exercise and Flexibility

Most men and women in their 20s should find it fairly easy to touch their toes without bending their knees. At 30, they will probably be a few inches short of the floor, at 40 six or seven inches, at 60 the whole idea may seem ridiculous. That's what the aging process does, particularly if we accelerate it by ignoring the need for elasticity of muscles and ligaments.

Men and women of 20 *should* find it fairly easy to touch their toes. Increasingly, they do not. Constant sitting in front of a television set develops the "TV legs syndrome" – a shortening of the hamstrings (the muscles of the back of the thigh) and a loss of flexibility of the lower back, giving them the range of movement of a 40-year-old.

Even children are affected. According to the standard Kraus-Weber test of flexibility, youngsters age 6 to 12 should be able to touch their palms to the floor. Tests in a Toronto suburb a few years ago produced failure rates of 75 per cent for boys and 58 per cent for girls. The aging process is really starting young. Surveys indicate many children spend some 21 hours a week or more in front of the TV set; TV legs are just one symptom of what's happening to them physically. George Bernard Shaw once remarked that youth was such a great thing it was a pity to waste it on children. Now it appears even the children are wasting it.

A flexible body is just as important to the average person as it is to the gymnast or diver. Aches, pains, inability to move easily, and chronic fatigue are all symptoms of poor flexibility. The flexible body bends, rather than breaks; it absorbs shocks more easily and is thus a protection against injury.

Flexibility is one of the first physical capabilities to leave you when you become sedentary. By decreasing the sinovial fluid which lubricates the joints, inactivity affects their range of movement and causes aching and stiffness. You start to feel old before you should because physically you are getting "old", even if the calendar doesn't say so.

The great characteristic of youth is free, easy, and unrestricted movement; when you've lost it, you've lost your youth.

The chief problem is maintaining the proper tone, efficiency and elasticity of all the various ligaments which hold the body structure together. These tremendously strong "holding wires" composed of elastic connective tissue have the ability to contract, and often do after activity. Aching joints and muscles after a hard day on your feet, or after a stiff workout, may be due in part to shortened ligaments. If they have become shortened through inactivity, after a few years even mild activity may cause you to creak a bit. Further, posture may suffer – those ligaments won't let you stand up straight.

Ligaments can also be stretched too far. For example, when you sprain an ankle, you stretch the ligament past its ability to snap back and return the ankle bones to their proper position. There may even be some tearing, requiring surgical repair in more serious cases. A short, tense ligament is more easily stretched since its lack of elasticity does not permit it to move very far. It may then become a loose ligament – one which does not hold the bones together tightly enough. Certain exercises such as vigorous deep knee bends may even contribute to this condition; there is lack of agreement among the experts on this point, however.

Full flexibility involves muscles and tendons as well as the ligaments. Fortunately, flexibility is a recoverable commodity, as Chapter 4 will show you.

Exercise and Metabolism

Some diet experts like to quote the number of calories you must use up to get rid of a pound of fat (about 3,500). This is roughly equivalent to chopping wood for seven hours or jogging 35 miles, they tell you. This is true as far as it goes – but don't let such statistics mislead you as to the value of exercise in a weight reduction campaign.

There are at least two factors not included in this statistic:

1. The duration of exercise: you don't have to chop that wood all at once; you can do it in a day, a week, or a year and those 3,500 calories will still be used up. Thirty minutes of daily woodchopping continued for a year would eliminate 26 pounds of fat.

2. The positive effect of exercise on your metabolism which governs the rate at which you burn up those calories.

What is metabolism? Basal metabolism has been defined as the irreducible minimum amount of energy required to keep up the life process. It is highest at birth, decreasing as you get older. This is one reason why you may suddenly start to put on weight even though your diet remains unchanged.

The metabolic rate increases during exercise; you expend more energy (burn up calories), the amount depending on the vigorousness of the activity. But here is the dividend: your metabolic rate doesn't fall back to normal as soon as you stop exercising. The oxidative recovery processes keep on working in the body after exercise stops, particularly after hard muscular effort, and so the metabolic rate takes some time to return to normal.

Dr. Herbert deVries found that the resting metabolic rate could be anywhere from 7.5 to 28 per cent higher 4 hours after a vigorous workout. Dr. T. K. Cureton measured increases which persisted for as long as 2 days, at which time another round of exercise would be required.

It is clear that the best way to prevent the slowdown of the metabolic process and its companion burden of extra fat is physical activity. The kind of exercise that has the greatest effect is vigorous enough to increase the heart rate to the target zone (page 61) – brisk walking, jogging, squash, tennis, cycling, swimming – and should last for at least 30 minutes.

Exercise and Appetite

Some individuals trying to lose weight avoid exercise because they are afraid it will increase their appetite. Wrong!

Inactivity, rather than exercise, is likely to cause overeating. Overeating, simply defined, means taking in more calories than you burn up. The unused calories are stored as fat.

Our appetite is controlled by a mechanism known as the "appestat". Dr. Jean Mayers, one of the world's foremost experts on nutrition, has found that this mechanism does not function properly in two instances: 1. when there is too little activity appetite tends to increase and, 2. when there is too much (reaching physical exhaustion levels) appetite tends to decrease.[3]

In their book, *Slim Chance in a Fat World*,[4] Dr. Richard B. Stuart and Barbara Davis point out that exercise before a meal will frequently decrease appetite. Further, they say, exercise helps to alleviate the tension and boredom which sometimes create a psychological need to overeat.

There is another plus for exercise: you don't have to restrict your calorie intake quite so drastically in order to lose weight. Regular exercise will burn up enough calories so that you can eat extra food to take the edge off that craving which places such a heavy load on your willpower.

Severe cutbacks in caloric intake – crash diets – without exercise may also be ineffective because the basal metabolism reacts to starvation by slowing down. Weight loss will be faster if a higher metabolism is maintained through exercise.

Exercise and Your Bones

How, you may ask, can exercise possibly affect your bones, apart from the risk of damage if you drop a barbell on your foot? Exercise helps to prevent osteoporosis, a progressive disease which makes bones porous, weak, and brittle. It may set in as early as age 30, but usually it doesn't manifest itself until the 60s. Osteoporosis is more widespread than you might realize. Medical evidence indicates that one out of four women past menopause suffers from some form of this disease.

Our bones are composed of calcium, phosphate, and carbonate, cemented together with a substance called collagen. Osteoporosis is caused by loss of some of the mineral and collagen, leaving the bones pitted like a sponge. Inactivity can affect the rate at which bone resorption takes place. Experiments were conducted on a group of young people who remained in bed with their bodies encased in plaster casts. Calcium began to be excreted within a few days, indicating that bone depletion was taking place.

How can exercise forestall osteoporosis? First, physical activity stimulates the formation of new bone tissue (osteoblast) since the pulling action of the muscles and tendons on the bones causes the bones to grow and become stronger to meet the stress of exercise. Second, the bones contain tiny blood vessels through which nutrients for health and growth are transported, and exercise stimulates the flow of blood through these vessels.

The back and the hips are among the most vulnerable areas for osteoporosis, so walking, jogging, and swimming as well as rhythmic arm and shoulder exercises are valuable preventive measures, particularly for older people. Most types of exercise which increase muscular strength and cardiovascular fitness are beneficial for the average person.

And don't forget the role of nutrition. Calcium, vitamin D (which controls the process governing formation of bone tissue), and phosphorus are important. Since we consume a lot of meat and soft drinks, we probably get far more phosphorus than we need and not enough calcium. Dairy products are high in calcium; so are leafy green vegetables, nuts, soybeans, molasses, and figs; while Vitamin D is present in sunshine, liver, eggs, sardines, salmon, and is often added to milk. Medical evidence indicates that most adults obtain sufficient vitamin D for their needs, but that growing children frequently do not.

Exercise and Cigarettes

Exercise will not reduce the risk of cancer and many other health hazards; but, surprisingly enough, smokers can achieve quite a high oxygen uptake level through regular exercise.

Oxygen uptake represents the efficiency with which we extract oxygen from the air at the lungs and feed it to working muscles. Smokers, according to tests done on a large group of people ranging in age from 18 to 65 who averaged 25 cigarettes a day, do have a lower oxygen uptake than non-smokers. In this particular study, the smokers averaged about 28 millilitres per minute per kilogram of bodyweight, while non-smokers tested out at 31 ml/kg/min.

After three months of training, the smokers had improved their scores by 18 per cent, the non-smokers by 19 per cent. This ratio was sustained as the study program continued; on the average, smokers were never able to achieve equal status. A similar trend was noticed in heart performance scores (resting, standing, after-activity and recovery pulse rates) and in blood pressure scores.[5]

The study indicated that the longer the person had smoked, and the more heavily he or she had smoked, the lower the initial VO_2 score was likely to be and the longer it took to improve it.

The significant factor is this: smoking damages the individual's most important fitness asset, the ability to utilize oxygen. Regular training, however, can help the individual recoup a great deal of this loss, an important fact to remember. If you smoke, it's even more essential that you exercise.

Exercise and Aging

Gerontologists say that the average person's productive adult life can be extended past the present average by some 20 per cent through regular physical activity of the proper type. What an individual can do in his or her 50s, he or she should be able to do at 70.

Dr. Herbert deVries of California, who is one of the leaders in this field, has pointed out that old people respond extremely well to exercise. It gives them renewed energy, a definite lift in morale, and reduces their physiological age.

In-depth research is still needed to show the specific physical declines caused by aging, but recent work strongly indicates that levels which are now accepted should not be. Those who live longest are those who refuse to accept the idea of aging. They retain their interest in their hobbies, the world around them, and their physical capabilities, and they do something about them. They ignore the warnings of those who say it's time to slow down and take things easy.

We tend to forget that the brain has arteries too. If we allow the circulation to deteriorate as we get older, not only is the supply of blood *to* the brain diminished, but also the flow *within* the brain. To function efficiently, it needs oxygen. Poor circulation deprives it of an adequate supply.

Clinical psychologists at the Veterans Administration Hospital in Buffalo, N.Y., placed senile patients in pressurized chambers called hyperbarics, and supplied them with pure oxygen at above-atmospheric pressure for three hours a day. After 51 days, their scores on standard memory tests had improved appreciably. Unfortunately, when the special oxygen treatment was discontinued, the patients returned to their previous levels in a short time.

This is just one more demonstration why regular physical activity, which keeps circulation levels in good shape, becomes more and more important as you grow older.

MOTIVATION FOR A NEW LIFE STYLE

How Long Does It Take?

How long it takes is up to you. How much time are you prepared to spend, and how fit do you want to get? Three days a week is enough, if your program is well-organized. Four or five is better. Seven is wonderful, but it shouldn't be all programmed work. Organize your life style so that you have some sort of physical activity every day. If your fitness levels are low, you'll have to be prepared to spend about 45 minutes at least three times a week on special exercises for those areas which self-testing has shown to be seriously below par.

Some programs advertise fitness in virtually no time with no effort. There is some evidence that exercising for five minutes at 90 per cent of maximum heart rate will improve cardiovascular endurance, but work at this intensity is not advisable for the average untrained individual, especially anyone over 30. The latest information from the American College of Sports Medicine, the Canadian Department of Health and Welfare, and the Soviet Union is that 15 minutes of vigorous exercise at 70 to 85 per cent of maximum heart rate is required for a good training effect, and this is for the heart-circulatory system alone. It doesn't take into account the special exercises you'll need for improving your own particular weaknesses.

Besides, most of the quickie fitness programs are misleading because they guide you subtly into heavier and heavier workloads. That's good, of course, because you're developing a new life style, and that's essential if you are to get fit and stay fit without placing insuperable demands on your willpower.

You'll need supplementary fitness activities as well – games, walking, swimming, dancing, gardening, anything you enjoy. You'll have to look for ways to increase activity, not avoid it – even if it's only walking briskly over to your TV set to change programs rather than using remote control. Why ride when you can walk? Why walk slowly when you can walk briskly? Why take an elevator when climbing stairs is a valuable fitness activity (in moderation, to start)? Why suffer through crash diets when possibly all you need is to increase your calorie burn up by 200 calories per day and to decrease your intake by the same amount? Why suffer excess tension and anxiety when relaxation is a physical skill you can learn?

Why feel old when it's almost as easy to feel young – and a lot more rewarding? And why wait until tomorrow or next week or next year when it's as simple as getting up from your chair right now and starting a fitness campaign by walking or cycling briskly around the block?

Why Many Fitness Campaigns Fail

Most fitness campaigns fail for the simple reason that they're not really fitness campaigns at all – they're rather aimless attempts to do something about physical shortcomings. There are no long-range objectives, and no short-term goals. The individual doesn't know what level of fitness he or she has to start with, has no idea whether useful progress is being made, no motivation to keep going, and little concept of where the road leads apart from a general desire to go "somewhere".

Like Stephen Leacock's hero, all too often we fling ourselves on a horse and ride madly off in all directions. No wonder so many people start their program enthusiastically, and then gradually peter out.

There are two things you must accept before you start your fitness campaign.

1. You will have to change your life style. If you are unfit, it is because your life style is too inactive. You must be prepared not only to embark on an exercise program and to adjust your nutrition pattern, but also to become more active generally. You don't have to go to extremes. Even a half-hour of extra walking at a brisk pace every day will work wonders. Do what you like, but do *something*, and do it regularly. Break your sedentary pattern of living. Look for fitness opportunities in everything you do. It's easy,

once you get the knack.

2. You will have to plan your fitness campaign. Know how fit you want to get, and decide on your short-term goals. This is essential for personal motivation.

Suppose, for example, that you are a keen gardener. You would accomplish little without a plan. You have to know what you are going to grow and where. Your long-range objective is to produce the garden you've planned and visualized in your mind. You do not achieve this by pottering around. You set short-term goals: "Today I am going to dig compost into the vegetable patch"; "Today I am going to plant the roses." If you dug and planted at random, chances are you'd soon lose interest.

Fitness is like that too. You don't get much done unless you know the sort of body you want to "grow" and have a day-to-day plan of how to go about it.

Start by testing your present fitness levels, and by relating the results to certain standards which you will attempt to reach and pass. The reasons and techniques for testing are more fully explained in Chapter 3.

Willpower is difficult to exercise if you haven't got any. Flab is mental as well as physical. Fortunately, willpower is like a muscle: it grows with training. As habits change, life gets easier. Sometimes, of course, you will have to force yourself. Make up your mind to do this, too, before starting your program. Be prepared to psych yourself up as an athlete does before a game or practice.

A final thought about mental attitude and willpower. People seem to fall into two categories. Some intensify problems and tasks ("This is going to be difficult; this really hurts; I'll never manage it."). Others diminish difficulties by regarding them as unimportant and easily conquered.

How do you handle your problems? Learn to accept life's chores cheerfully and attack them with vigor and enthusiasm.

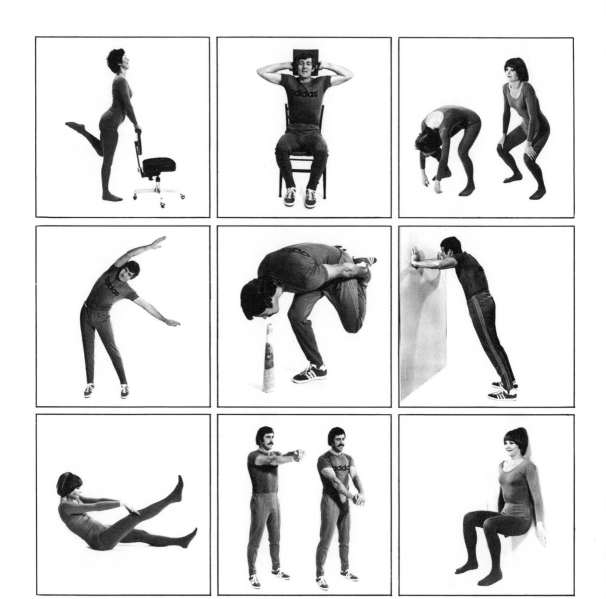

Fitness and Exercise

3

What Shape Are You Really In?

DEFINING YOUR PROBLEMS AND SETTING YOUR GOALS

In many ways, physical fitness is like money in the bank. It is a tangible reward for effort. Like all rewards it must be visible – you must know how much of it you have, otherwise you will lack both a sense of achievement and the motivation to acquire more.

This is why self-testing is a vital ingredient of any fitness program. Measurable improvement becomes your bank account; making it grow becomes your objective.

Lack of visible success is one major reason for the failure of so many fitness programs. After months of effort, you have no real indication of what you have managed to achieve. There may be a certain sense of wellbeing; you may be able to do some things which were beyond your capability when you started – but you still don't know exactly how much "money" you have in the bank. You cannot be sure that you are solving your real fitness problems.

Suppose, for example, that you are a jogger. You may stick at it long enough to run two miles at a fairly good pace. But, like the distance runner who has not had a time trial, you cannot be positive that you're doing exactly what you set out to do. What,

specifically, have you done for your cardiovascular system? How much more efficient has it become? Have you reached a point where you should be considering a shift in emphasis to provide more work on your flexibility? What is your arm and leg strength? How is your abdominal fitness? How do you rate overall?

Without testing, there's no real way of knowing. The effort you are expending may start to seem rather pointless. That's why a lot of people give up.

Define the Problem

Before you start a program of self-improvement, you need to isolate your problems. Then you can find the solutions scientifically, emphasizing what will help you most. Testing can help you to design a program that will suit your physical needs, your personality, and the time you have available.

For example, you may find that your flexibility levels are generally good, with the exception of the backs of your thighs. (You probably spend a lot of time sitting down.) Lack of hamstring flexibility can make gardening or even tying your shoes difficult, so spend some time on exercises for this area. But don't bother wasting too much effort on exercises to increase the flexibility of your upper body if tests show you already have it.

Or you may be one of those rare individuals with extremely good heart-wind fitness. A lot of running, bicycling, or other cardiovascular activity is probably not what you really need. Unless you're planning to become a competitive athlete, do enough for maintenance purposes. Shift the emphasis in your fitness program to something you do need — perhaps strength in the arms and shoulders, or the abdomen.

We are born with specific physical characteristics — organic efficiency, numbers and types of muscle fibers, for example — which predispose us toward certain activities and away from others. Heavily-muscled individuals seldom become distance runners simply because their body channels them in another direction, and consequently that direction is where their preferences will lie.

People with good heart-wind fitness prefer activities which develop heart-wind fitness; strong people like to do strength exercises. Conversely, weak people usually dislike strength exercises; people who get out of breath easily try to avoid jogging or other activities which make them puff and pant.

When we start a fitness program, we tend to avoid those activities or exercises which will strengthen our weaknesses. If we play to our strengths, our fitness program may be less effective than it should be because it may create an unbalanced organism. We can't separate the fitness of one area from the fitness of another; to be totally fit, we must condition the total organism uniformly.

Set Goals and Objectives

In addition to knowing your problems, you must have some idea of where you are going — an objective. You need short-term goals as well as long-term goals, even if they're only simple ones.

For example, your long-term objective might be to lower your standing heart rate to 60 from its present 84. Your short-term objective might be to break 80. Once this is achieved, set further short-term objectives until you reach the sub-60 level.

Both the fitness acolyte and the super athlete have a need for achievement, and achievement must be measured in personal terms. Testing provides a yardstick with which to measure progress. Testing motivates, for when we see the results of our physical activity, we are likely to persevere.

As another example, your long-term objective could be to run a mile under seven minutes. Make your short-term objective nine minutes. Gradually bring your short-term objectives closer to that seven minute mark; then drop the seven to six, and start over again.

It is important to know where you're going and to *want* to get there. Your goal might be playing three hard sets of tennis without feeling tired or stiff, or swimming across the channel at the summer cottage, or lifting X number of pounds in your weight-lifting program, or skiing cross-country fast enough to keep up with the gang.

You don't achieve these objectives all at once; you travel step by step, relishing the pleasure of achieving each new plateau until you attain your goal.

When you've done that, set new goals and work to achieve those. All too often the complacent alternative — "I've done it, now I can sit back and rest" — leads us back to the old problems, and we have to start all over again.

TESTING YOUR FITNESS

The Testing Program

This testing program, which has been developed and refined over the years, is one which anyone can do at home without scientific equipment. It is not designed to give you a passing or failing mark, but to measure your physical capabilities in the most important areas relating to total fitness. It is designed to chart your progress and to show you where your exercise or activity emphasis should fall.

There are two things to remember. First, a fitness test is not a substitute for a medical examination. Discuss your planned fitness campaign with your doctor before you take the tests. Get his advice, especially on those tests which place a strain on your cardiovascular system. If you have a structural problem, such as weakness in the lower back, avoid or modify certain tests and exercises. These are indicated in Chapter 5.

Second, although these tests have been scientifically devised, they will not provide an exact measure of your physical status. This can only be done in a laboratory with expensive equipment and trained technicians. These tests will, however, give you a good indication of your level of fitness; will help you to work on your weak areas; and, most important, will show you where you stand now and how much you have progressed in two months or two years. Once you start getting into good shape, even on your own scale, you'll be well ahead of 80 per cent of the adult population.

These tests will not measure all the areas such as blood pressure and oxygen uptake which a physiologist would explore if you stepped into his lab. They will measure the most significant factors of fitness which can be tested easily at home.

In order to measure progress, it is important to keep a record of your performance in each test. Draw up a scoreboard similar to the one illustrated on page 52. Always record the date and such pertinent data as your weight and the type of program or activity (if any) which led up to the test. For example, if you have been doing a lot of gardening, or playing tennis, or cross-country skiing in the weeks prior to your test,

keep track of this fact. In this way you will be able to see the effects of each of these activities.

You might make this a family fitness campaign. Some of the tests and exercises require assistance, and there is certainly added pleasure and motivation when two or more people become involved in a common project. Never mind the loneliness of the long distance runner – the fitness buff can suffer the discouragement of isolation as well. It helps to know that you're not alone in your struggle.

Get your friends interested and arrange to meet in a different house once or twice a week for group fitness activities, in addition to your own sessions at home. The empathy of other people will help you through the rough patches and motivate you when you most require it – and vice versa.

One way to interest your friends is to try this testing program at a party – a challenge to see who's the fittest in each area (make sure there are no potential cardiac cases among them, and omit the heart-wind tests which could cause problems.) Chances are just about everybody will do poorly, at least in a number of areas; that in itself should challenge them to get involved, particularly if you discuss the implications of your common physical failures afterwards.

Common fitness weaknesses are:

Men: heart-wind, fat, flexibility

Women: fat, abdominal strength, flexibility

Boys: (pre-adolescent) strength, especially arm and abdominal area; (teenage) strength, flexibility, agility

Girls: (pre-adolescent) abdominal strength, agility, reaction time; (teenage) fat, strength

Some Guidelines

It's best to test yourself at approximately the same time every day. Heart rates and other factors vary from morning to night. It also stands to reason that if you've had an unusual amount of physical activity during the day – such as digging in the garden, or a long hike – your work capacity will be affected. Do your testing on an average day.

Make sure that at least two hours have elapsed since your last big meal. Resting heart rates will tend to be appreciably higher while you're digesting food, and you may feel lethargic if you have a full stomach while doing the tests. It's also a good idea to avoid smoking, or drinking tea or coffee for an hour before the test since they may affect heart performance.

Separate your tests as far as possible from the taking of medication, particularly tranquilizers or stimulants.

Those tests which are contraindicated for people with low back problems, suspected heart conditions, or high blood pressure have been noted. Don't do them without permission from your doctor. However, a particular weakness should be one of your priorities in selecting exercises for your fitness program. While certain exercises may be contraindicated, there are others which you can do safely and which will help your particular problem.

Taking Your Pulse

From time to time you'll be required to take your pulse rate as a measure of activity intensity and/or recovery from effort. There are a number of ways it can be done.

It's popular in physical-education circles to use the carotid artery – the artery located just in front of the large neck muscle under the jawbone. You can find it by tracing a line with your fingers from the front of the ear down over the jaw, where you'll feel the edge of the muscle alongside the throat. The pulse is quite strong there.

If you are using this method, be careful not to press too hard or to place your thumb at the same time on the second carotid artery on the other side of the neck, since you may reduce blood flow to the brain. This can cause dizziness or blackouts. For the same reason, do not palpate (massage) the artery, as this may interfere with the flow of messages between the brain and the heart.

Probably the safest and simplest method is taking the radial pulse in the wrist. Always use your fingers, since the thumb has a small pulse of its own and may give you an "echo" effect.

Hold the left arm level with the palm open and facing up. Place the other hand underneath and curl the fingers around at wrist-watch level, probing for the pulse on the thumb-side of the prominent tendons which run down the center of the wrist. Press heavily and release gradually until you sense the pulse under the fingertips. With a little practice you'll be able to touch the spot every time.

Count your pulse beat for 15 seconds rather than for the full minute, and multiply by four to get the number of beats per minute. There's a reason for this. One of the measures of heart efficiency is its ability to recover from effort. As you get fit, the recovery period should become shorter and shorter. If you count the pulse rate for a full minute, the heart will be beating much slower at the end of the minute than it was at the beginning, and you'll get an inaccurate reading.

For example, in the step test you want to know the difference between resting pulse rate and post-exertion pulse rate. Immediately after your test it might be 150 beats per minute. But a minute later, it might be down to 120 or lower, so counting the pulse for 15 seconds and multiplying by four would be the only way to get an accurate reading.

You may lose or add a beat this way, since it's hard to be spot on with a 15-second check, but the error over the full minute will be only four and that's not significant for our purposes.

16 Tests of Fitness

To determine your scores in the following tests, consult the table on page 50.

1. CRAMPTON TEST

Lie quietly on back on floor for 3 minutes. Take pulse (refer to instructions above for correct procedure). Stand up *slowly*, wait 10 seconds and take pulse again. Calculate difference between lying and standing pulse rate.

Measures: Simple heart performance.

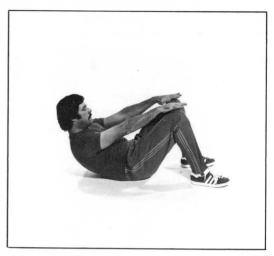

▲
3. ABDOMINAL HOLD

Lie on floor on back, feet flat on floor about hip-width apart with knees bent at right angles. Place hands on tops of thighs, arms straight. Keeping arms straight, raise upper body until fingertips reach knees (shoulders will be about 12 inches from the floor). Try to keep the back straight and to breathe normally; do not hold breath. Record in seconds how long you can hold this position. If you are overweight, you may find it necessary to hook your feet under a couch or dresser, or have someone hold them down. Be sure to curl the body slowly down to the floor, especially if you have low back or neck problems.

Measures: Strength of abdominal muscles.

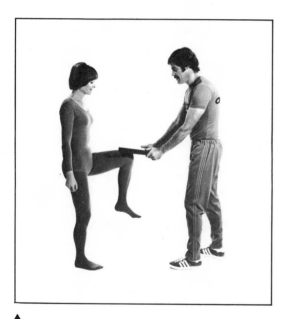

▲
2. FAST KNEE LIFT

Secure a book or magazine in front of you at hip height or have a partner hold it for you. Lift alternate knees as fast as possible to touch book. It's similar to high-knee running on the spot except that one foot must always remain on the floor. Count number of times you can touch book in 10 seconds.

Measures: Speed of muscular movement.

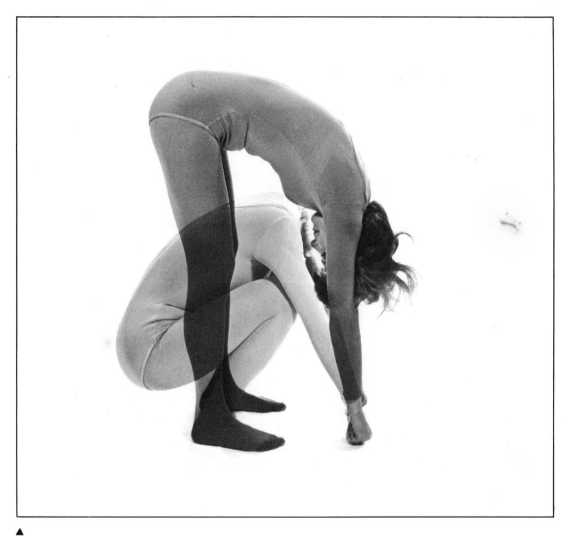

▲
4. BACK THIGH STRETCH

With feet hip-width apart, squat on floor with fists just in front of your toes. Keep heels down and head tucked in looking between legs. Slowly try to straighten your legs while keeping both heels and fists on floor. Head should remain down so that you are still looking between your legs. If unsuccessful, move fists out 3 inches at a time until you can straighten your legs. Measure distance between toes and fists.

Measures: Flexibility of back thigh muscles.

5. STANDING BROAD JUMP

Measure your height, then make 2 marks on the floor that distance apart. Stand with feet hip-width apart, toes on first mark. Jump as far past second mark as you can, landing on both feet. (Try to absorb shock of landing in knees, not back.) Measure distance from point where heels touch down to the second mark. If you fail to reach the mark, your distance is calculated as a minus for purposes of scoring.

Measures: Muscle power.

42

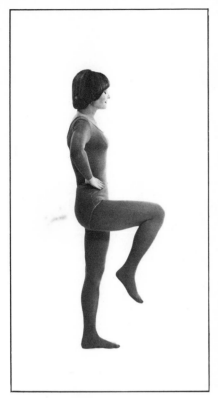

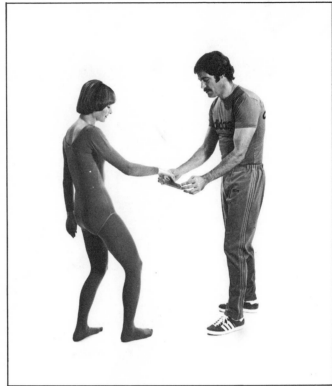

6. STORK STAND

First, stand with hands on hips, feet hip-width apart, eyes open. Raise right knee to hip height and hold for 5 seconds. Return foot to floor and repeat with left knee. Now repeat the same movements with eyes closed. The supporting foot must not move, hands must remain on hips, the knee must not drop below hip height, and the eyes must remain closed all through the movement (which includes the transition from right to left). Only one attempt is allowed—no second chances.

Scoring

Eyes open, right 5 seconds	2
Eyes open, left 5 seconds	2
Eyes closed, right 5 seconds	2
Eyes closed, transition	2
Eyes closed, left 5 seconds	2
Total points	10

Measures: Balance (kinesthetic sense).

7. RULER DROP

Have a partner hold a ruler horizontally at your waist height, supporting it at the ends with his fingertips. Place your open right hand directly over ruler but not touching it. Have your partner drop ruler without warning. Try to catch it with right hand before it reaches floor. Do twice with right hand, twice with left hand, twice with both hands. Record total number of catches. Hint: stand with knees bent and one foot slightly advanced.

Measures: Reaction time.

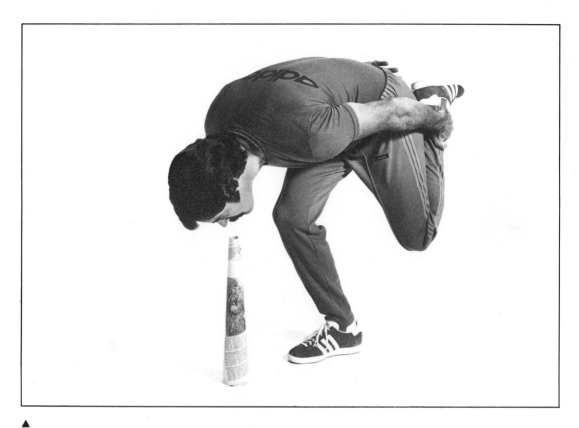

▲

8. PAPER PICK UP

Make 3 cones from rolled-up newspapers, 20,
15, and 10 inches tall. Stand them in a line
on the floor in front of you. Raise your non-
dominant leg behind you, bending it at the
knee, and clasp it with both hands. (Your
non-dominant leg is the one with which you
would *not* kick a ball.) Standing on the
dominant leg, bend over and pick up the 20-
inch cone with your teeth and return to
starting position without losing balance. If
successful, score 4. You are allowed two
tries. Move to the 15-inch cone and try again.
Score 4 more points if you succeed. Score an
additional 6 points if you pick up the 10-inch
cone.

> **Measures:** Flexibility, strength, and
> balance.

> **Contraindicated for:** High blood
> pressure.

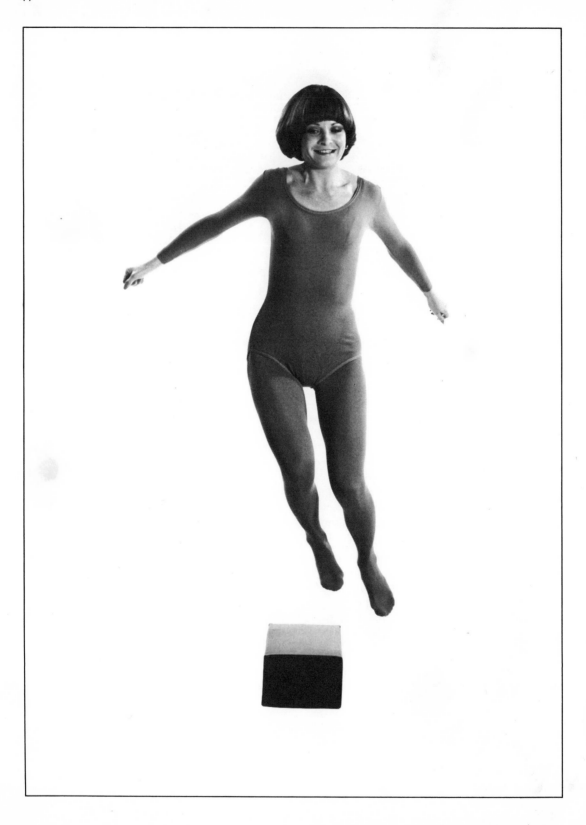

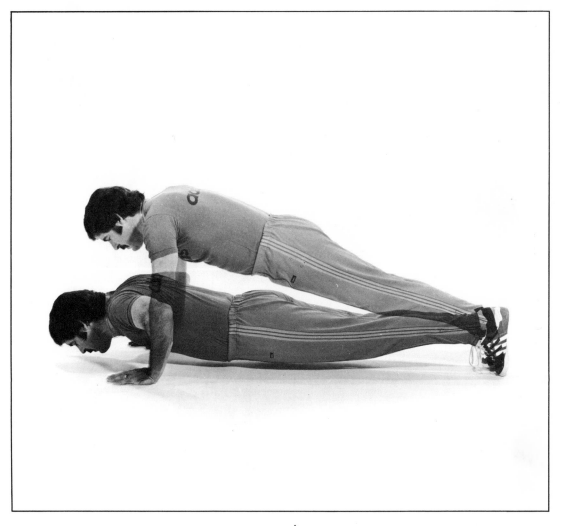

◄ 9. AGILITY JUMP

▲
10. PUSH-UP HOLD

Pile books on the floor to a height of approximately 4 to 6 inches, one on top of the other. Stand beside them with feet together. Jump sideways back and forth over the books as fast as you can, counting the number of times you clear them in 10 seconds. Attempt to keep the feet together throughout.

Measures: Agility.

Lie face down on the floor with hands directly under shoulders. Do a push-up (men from the feet, women from the knees), keeping the body straight. Now lower yourself until your elbows are bent at right angles. Record the number of seconds you can hold this position without allowing the body to drop or sag. Do not hold breath.

Measures: Strength of arms and upper body.

Contraindicated for: High blood pressure.

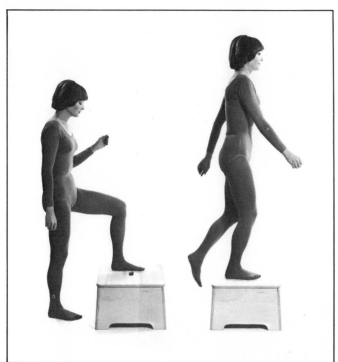 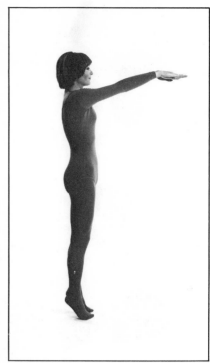

▲

▲

11. CHAIR STEP UP

For this test you will need a chair or box about 16 inches high. Relax in a chair and take your pulse rate. Make sure you are recovered from any previous exertion so that your resting rate is not higher than it should be. Start test by stepping up and down from chair or box at the rate of 1 step every 3 seconds. To step properly, start with your left foot, bring right foot up beside it and then step down again with left foot first, then right. Continue for 2 minutes, at which time you should have done about 40 step ups. You may change the lead leg after 20 step ups.

Now relax in a chair for 1 minute and take your pulse again. Calculate the difference between post- and pre-step pulse rates to obtain score.

Measures: Cardiorespiratory fitness.

Contraindicated for: Heart/circulatory conditions.

12. DIVER'S HOLD

Take off your shoes and stand with your feet together, hands at sides and eyes closed. Raise arms to shoulder level in front and at the same time come up on your toes as high as possible, like a diver. Hold for 1 minute. Your score is the number of seconds you can hold position without losing balance or opening eyes.

Measures: Balance and general motor ability.

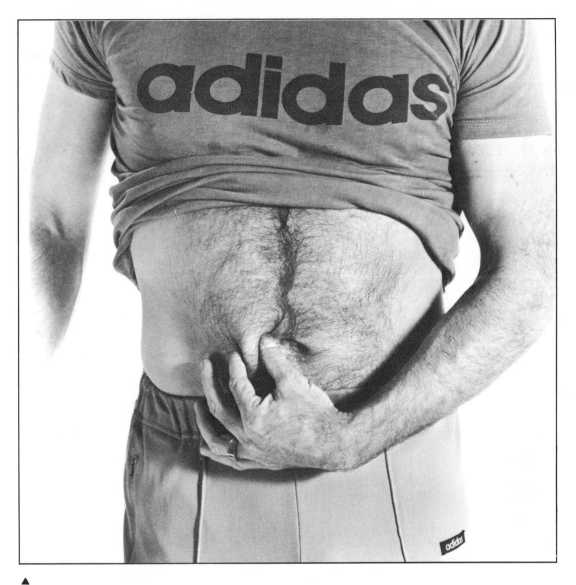

▲

13. PINCH TEST

Using thumb and forefinger, pinch up the skin and underlying fat on your abdomen just beside the navel in a vertical roll. Roll finger and thumb together slightly to make sure you haven't pinched up a bit of the underlying muscle. Measure fat thickness carefully with a ruler.

Measures: Abdominal fat (an indication of overall fat content).

48

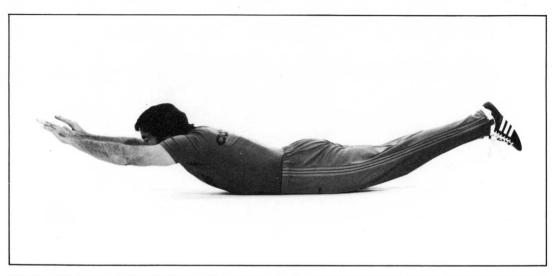

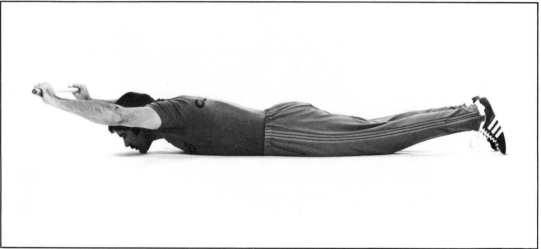

▲
14. ROCKER LIFT HOLD

Lie on stomach with your arms stretched out in front of you. Raise arms, upper body, and legs as far from floor as possible and hold as long as you can (maximum of 1 minute for men, 35 seconds for women). Knees must be kept as straight as possible. Test ends as soon as either arms or legs touch floor. Score is holding time in seconds.

Measures: Back muscle strength.

Contraindicated for: Low back and neck problems.

▲
15. SHOULDER FLEX

Lie face down on the floor. Using a slightly wider than shoulder-width grip, hold a stick or broom handle at arm's length in front of you. Raise arms as high as possible with elbows and wrists straight and chin on floor. Have your partner measure elevation of stick.

Measures: Shoulder flexibility.

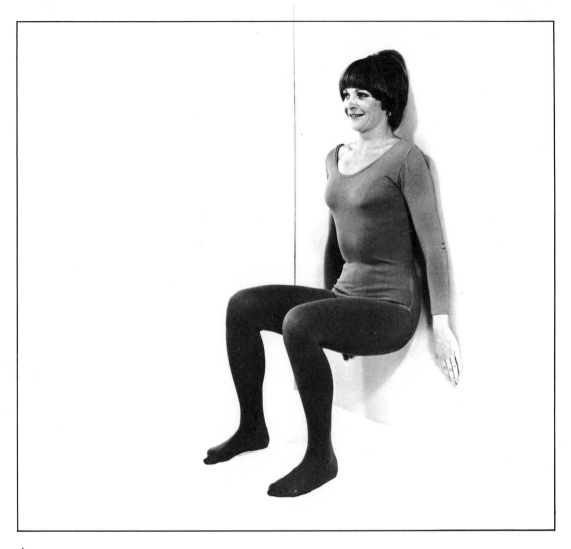

▲
16. SKI SIT

With back against wall, lower yourself into a sitting position by sliding down and moving feet out so that the heels remain directly under the knees. Your thighs should be parallel to the floor with the knees bent at right angles. The hands may not be used for assistance. Your score is the number of seconds you can hold this position.

Measures: Strength of leg muscles.

Contraindicated for: High blood pressure.

FITNESS TEST SCORING TABLE

POINTS SCORED ►	30	25	20	18	16	14	12	10	8	6	4	2	0 (UNSUCCESSFUL OR DID NOT ATTEMPT)
1. Crampton Test	0	1-2	3-4	5-6	7-8	9-10	11-12	13-14	15-16	17-18	19-20	21+	
2. Fast Knee Lift							40+	35-39	30-34	25-29	20-24	0-19	
3. Abdominal Hold — Men			61+	54-60	47-53	40-46	32-39	25-31	17-24	10-16	5-9	0-4	
Abdominal Hold — Women			37+	32-36	28-31	24-27	19-23	15-18	10-14	6-9	3-5	0-2	
4. Back Thigh Stretch					0	0-4	4-8	8-12	12-16	16-20	20-24	25+	
5. Standing Broad Jump			21+	16-20	12-16	8-12	4-8	0-4	0 to -4	-4 to -8	-8 to -12	-12 or less	
6. Stork Stand								10	8	6	4	2	
7. Ruler Drop							6	5	4	3	2	1	
8. Paper Pick Up						10"			15"		20"		
9. Agility Jump					22+	19-21	16-18	13-15	10-12	7-9	4-6	1-3	
10. Push-Up Hold — Men–Feet			61+	54-60	47-53	40-46	32-39	25-31	17-24	10-16	5-9	0-4	
Push-Up Hold — Women–Knees			37+	32-36	28-31	24-27	19-23	15-18	10-14	6-9	3-5	0-2	
11. Chair Step Up	0	1-5	6-10	11-15	16-20	21-25	26-30	31-35	36-40	41-45	46-50	51+	
12. Diver's Hold					61+	51-60	41-50	31-40	21-30	11-20	6-10	0-5	
13. Pinch Test		1/4 or less	1/4-1/2	1/2-3/4	3/4-1	1-1 1/4	1 1/4-1 1/2	1 1/2-1 3/4	1 3/4-2	2-2 1/4	2 1/4-2 1/2	2 1/2+	
14. Rocker Lift Hold — Men			61+	54-60	47-53	40-46	32-39	25-31	17-24	10-16	5-9	0-4	
Rocker Lift Hold — Women			37+	32-36	28-31	24-27	19-23	15-18	10-14	6-9	3-5	0-2	
15. Shoulder Flex					18-20	16-18	14-16	12-14	10-12	8-10	4-8	0-9	
16. Ski Sit — Men			90+	80-89	70-79	60-69	50-59	40-49	30-39	20-29	10-18	0-9	
Ski Sit — Women			60+	53-59	47-52	41-46	35-40	29-34	23-28	17-22	10-16	0-9	

How to Use the Scoring Table

Each test is weighted according to its value for total fitness. For example, because heart-wind fitness is far more important to you than balance, it is possible to score a maximum of 30 in the 2 tests which measure heart-wind fitness, while 10 is the top score for balance.

You'll note that maximum scores vary throughout the 16 tests in the table: a possible 25 for minimum fat excess, 20 for abdominal and leg strength and so on down to 12 for muscle speed and 10 for balance. These maximums will be reflected in your "fitness profile" when you are deciding your fitness priorities.

To find your score, perform the test and note the column where the result falls in the table. Look to the top of the column for the score your performance has earned. For example, a difference of 11 to 12 in your resting and standing heart rates in the Crampton Test would earn 12.

When all the tests are completed, your total score will be the measure of your overall fitness. Although it will not reflect specific strengths and weaknesses, your total score will be useful. It will give you a baseline against which to measure your general progress during your fitness campaign, and so provide an objective; it is motivational. The average, untrained 30- to 40-year-old who has a fairly sedentary life style will probably score around the halfway mark or slightly lower in each test for a total of about 165. The 40- to 50-year-old can expect to drop a column in the scoring table, and the 50- to 60-year-old yet another column.

You will find that your aptitudes and activities are reflected in your highest and lowest scores. For example, a skier in season may test out well in leg and abdominal strength and still do badly in heart-wind performance. On the other hand, a person who does a lot of swimming or jogging may have good heart-wind scores but be low in back-thigh flexibility and agility.

A well-conditioned athlete should score 270 or better, a fit individual in the 30 to 40 age bracket around 240.

While one objective of your fitness program is to improve your overall score, your specific targets will be the top priority areas: heart-wind fitness, abdominal strength, fat content, arm and leg strength. Scores in the tests for which highest marks are awarded are the most significant because they measure these priorities.

A score of 8 for agility and 10 in the Crampton test of heart performance, for example, would tell you that you should emphasize heart-wind exercises and pay only moderate attention to agility drills. Heart performance is a high priority area, agility is not. Your score of 10 for heart performance gives you 33-1/3 per cent of maximum; your 8 in agility is 50 per cent. It is your standing in relation to maximum score that is significant, not the score itself. Keep this in mind when establishing your priorities.

The objective is to increase your rating in each category as much as you can. Success will depend on time, age, and inclination. It is unlikely, for example, that anyone but a trained athlete will score a maximum 30 in the chair step up. But 20 is not out of reach for people in their 50s if they get enough cardiovascular activity and are not overweight.

Similarly, you should try to reach 18 in the pinch test, 16 in abdominal strength and the push-up hold and 12 in shoulder flexibility.

As you grow older, your capabilities will decrease, more in some areas than in others. For example, endurance and muscle speed tend to diminish more quickly than strength.

It should be mentioned again that all these scores are arbitrary measures of fitness. Scientific measurement in a testing laboratory would be required to indicate your exact fitness in each area. For your requirements, however, the testing you do at home will be more than adequate. It will indicate your progress in each area in relation to your starting level.

A final note. In some of these tests a skill

YOUR FITNESS PROFILE

DATE _____ WT. _____ NO. OF WORKOUTS SINCE LAST TESTING

INITIAL TEST _____

1ST RETEST _____

2nd RETEST _____

3rd RETEST _____

TEST RESULTS

# Test	Measures	Max. Score	Initial Score	% of Max.	1st Retest Score	% of Max.	2nd Retest Score	% of Max.	3rd Retest Score	% of Max.
1 Crampton Test	Simple Heart Performance	30								
2 Fast Knee Lift	Speed of Muscular Movement	12								
3 Abdominal Hold	Strength of Abdominals	20								
4 Back Thigh Stretch	Flexibility of Back Thigh Muscles	16								
5 Standing Broad Jump	Muscle Power	20								
6 Stork Stand	Balance	10								
7 Ruler Drop	Reaction Time	12								
8 Paper Pick Up	Flexibility, Strength, Balance	14								
9 Agility Jump	Agility	16								
10 Push-Up Hold	Arm & Upper Body Strength	20								

No. / Test	Description	Value				
11 Chair Step Up	Cardiorespiratory Fitness	30				
12 Diver's Hold	Balance	16				
13 Pinch Test	Abdominal Fat – indicates overall fat content	25				
14 Rocker Lift Hold	Back Muscle Strength	20				
15 Shoulder Flex	Shoulder Flexibility	16				
16 Ski Sit	Legs – Muscle Strength	20				

Ranking Your Priorities		INITIAL		1ST RETEST		2ND RETEST		3RD RETEST	
		% of Max.	Rank	% of Max.	Rank	% of Max.	Rank	% of Max.	Rank
Cardiorespiratory Fitness	#11								
Simple Heart Performance	#1								
Fat Content	#13								
Strength of Abdominals	#3								
Arms & Upper Body	#10								
Legs	#8 #16								
Back	#14								
Flexibility of Back Thigh Muscles	#4								
Shoulders	#15								
Speed of Muscular Movement	#2								
Muscle Power	#5								
Motor Efficiency									
Balance	#8, #12, #6								
Reaction Time	#7								
Agility	#9								

factor is present. For example, you'll find that your scores in the ruler drop will improve if you keep your knees bent.

Do not let lack of success in such measures of motor skill and coordination as the balance test, ruler drop, and paper pick up discourage you. They rate fairly low in the total fitness picture, and will improve gradually without specific training as your fitness campaign progresses.

Determining Your Priorities

Before you can begin your program, you must establish priorities. To help you do this, a Fitness Profile has been provided (p. 52).

Take your score in each test and calculate what percent of maximum you have achieved. For example, 4 out of a possible 16 in the back thigh stretch would give you 25 per cent (4/16 x 100 = 25%). Your flexibility is one quarter of what it should be.

Note that certain priorities are listed above the line in Your Fitness Profile, while others relating to motor efficiency are below the line. Concentrate on the former; the others will improve as a function of increased fitness.

Now place a number 1 beside your lowest percentage above the line, a number 2 beside the second lowest, and so on. This will show you which areas are going to require the most attention when you are selecting exercises and activities for your fitness program. Keep in mind that certain factors are more important than others: a 50 per cent score in heart fitness is not as good as a 50 per cent score in back thigh flexibility because heart fitness rates a maximum of 30, while back thigh flexibility gets only 16 points.

The next chapter will tell you how to put together your program, based on these priorities, and will provide some sample programs for basic overall fitness with opportunity to add exercises for your specific problems.

You will find out if your programming has been accurate when the time comes for retesting after your first 24 workouts.

Retesting – Knowing That You've Made It Happen

When you have completed your testing and analyzed the results to establish priorities, you should move on to Chapter 4 which shows you how to organize a personal fitness program. After several workouts – 24 to start with – it will be time to retest. This is when you have a chance to measure your efforts: your improvement, or lack of it, becomes visible. Retesting provides the hard data which enable you to evaluate your program, make any necessary changes and move on to the next plateau.

This is a principal reason why you must keep a record of all your tests. Comparison with earlier results is not only a great motivator, but also gives you a year-long physiological profile. You may find that slight changes in emphasis are required according to the season. For example, if you're active in summer, but spend the winter in front of the television set, you may have to boost your heart-wind activity during the cold months to ward off a decline in that area.

It's a good idea to keep a fitness profile such as the one illustrated here. It should include the date, time of day, and weight at time of testing. Attach a copy of your exercise program to the card so you know what produced those particular results. Make notes about such factors as diet, recreational activities during that period, and frequency and number of workouts leading up to the test.

When you've completed each test, evaluate it carefully. Do you need more heart-wind activity? Should you have additional leg strength or abdominal work to create faster results? Are certain exercises too boring? Perhaps you should substitute alternative exercises for variety. Was self-motivation a problem? Perhaps less exercise activity and more recreational activity of a fitness type, such as swimming, badminton, or cycling, would be advisable to help you get through a rough period. Perhaps it's time to get some friends involved so you can have the motivational benefits of group activity.

As you can see, retesting not only provides visible results which show you how fast or how slowly you are moving toward your objective, it also allows you to be creative. An effective physical fitness program is not simply a monotonous, unvarying, military regime – it requires your mental involvement. This is the best way to maintain your motivation. When your mind switches off, your body stops working and you end up in front of the TV set again with your anxieties and high blood pressure.

You can retest as often as you want. But, like the kettle that refuses to boil when you keep an eye on it, results may take some time to show. There's no point in retesting "just to see how I'm coming along" after a few workouts. The lack of visible results may discourage you.

You should retest after your first 24 workouts, then after every 48 workouts. In this way, your gradual buildup of strength, flexibility and endurance will have a chance to become measureable.

4

How to Improve the Shape You're In

BASIC FITNESS PROGRAMS

Now that you have taken your tests and defined your priorities, you're ready to create your own fitness program. This chapter will help you get started.

There are a few things you should know before you begin. One is the basic format of an exercise program: the warm up, the body of the program in which strenuous exercises are separated by less vigorous ones so that you have brief recuperative periods, and the cool off. You should also be familiar with the law of repetitions which helps you decide how to progress, and you should know how to use your heart rate to monitor the intensity of your workout.

You should know something about strength and endurance, and how each is developed. You should also be aware of the circuit system of training, and how often to work out for best results.

Some of you may be a bit uncertain about the first step: creating a basic program. For this reason, three sample programs are provided as a model. They are in progressive phases so that, if you choose, you can work your way through and develop a good overall level of fitness before arriving at Phase 4 in which you alone are the programmer.

In each phase, just before the Cool Off, an asterisk designates that you may add further

exercises for your individual weaknesses or problems, as indicated by the results of your tests. (Choose these from the Exercise Bank in Chapter 5 or from Chapter 6, Special Problems.) This will help you get the feel of personal programming.

Testing will have indicated your overall fitness level, your so-called baseline. If it is low, Phase 1 may be a good place to start. However, your first workout may indicate that it is not sufficiently strenuous, in which case you can move quickly on to Phase 2 or even Phase 3. The latter, by the way, introduces you to circuit training.

Each exercise in Phase 1, 2 and 3 is numbered so you can locate it in the exercise "bank" provided in Chapter 5. Page numbers are given for exercises selected from other chapters. Start by doing the number of repetitions indicated in column 2 of the Phase outline, and build to the target figure in column 3. When you can handle this fairly easily, it's time to move up to the next phase.

Certain exercises in each phase may prove difficult. Even if you fail to reach your target in a particular exercise, you may move to the next phase, but take your problem with you, either by continuing the exercise in which you are "failing" or by scaling down the intensity of the corresponding exercise in the new phase. These problem exercises will tell you that you need more work in particular areas, and that you should include an extra drill or two from the exercise "bank" to help eliminate that weakness.

The speed at which you progress is up to you. Make sure that you do not try to do too much too soon. This is a common fault. Complaints from your muscles, joints and ligaments should be your guide. Better too little than too much, particularly if you are unfit.

PHASE 1

EXERCISE	START AT	BUILD TO	REST BETWEEN SETS
Warm Up			
Rag Doll Jog / 1	30 seconds–increase in 15-second increments	4 minutes	
Shoulder Shrug & Relax / 57	6 x 3 seconds		
Straight/Bent Arm Pull Back / p. 129	2 x 10 easy rhythm.	2 x 20	15 seconds
Seated Head/Knee Touch / p. 186	2 x 8		15 seconds
Program			
Rowing Push-Pull / 38	2 x 4 Start with 50% resistance.	2 x 8 maximum resistance	15 seconds
Quarter Squat / 2	3 x 10 Alternate with Ballet Squats (no. 12) every 3rd workout.	3 x 30	15 seconds
High Stretch and Relax / 40	6 x 3 seconds		
Stationary Walking / p. 102	30 seconds at a moderate pace. Add 15 seconds every few days, increasing speed.	2 minutes brisk pace	
Stomach Pull-In / 20	3 x 8 moderate tempo	3 x 20 brisk pace	15 seconds
Knee Push-Up / 31	3 x 4 Change hand position at half-way (apart/together).	3 x 12	15 seconds
Simulated Crawl / 39	2 x 20 easy rhythm		15 seconds
Step Up / 16	3 x 10 complete up and down steps. Change lead foot every 5 steps.	3 x 30	15 seconds
Torso Twist / 50	2 x 8	2 x 14	15 seconds
Lateral Side Bend / 48	2 x 10 easy rhythm	2 x 20	15 seconds
Bent Knee Sit Up / 22	3 x 4 easy pace	3 x 14 moderate pace	15 seconds
Lying Knee To Chest Tuck / 42	3 x 8		15 seconds
*Additional exercises of your choice			
Cool Off			
Rag Doll Jog / 1	30 seconds–increase in 15-second increments	4 minutes	
Arms Out, Up and Relax / 61	10 reps		
Seated Head/Knee Touch / p. 186	2 x 8		15 seconds
Monkey Slump / 64	6 reps		

PHASE 2

EXERCISE	START AT	BUILD TO	REST BETWEEN SETS
Warm Up			
Straddle Hop Arm Lift / 17	15 seconds at moderate pace, walk 15 seconds, repeat 4 times	x 6	Walk 15 seconds
Crucifix Collapse / 60	10 x 3 seconds		
Over Toe Reach / 45	8 x 5 seconds		
Willow Stretch / 51	2 x 4	2 x 8	15 seconds
Program			
Single Leg Jack-knife / 25	3 x 4	3 x 8	15 seconds
Fist Press-Pull / 37	2 x 4 moderate pressure	2 x 8 maximum resistance	15 seconds
Shadow Skipping / 18	1 minute–increase in 15-second increments. Increase speed and height of bounce.	5 minutes brisk pace	
Lateral Side Bend / 48	2 x 10	2 x 15	15 seconds
Arm Drill / 19	3 x 10 moderate pace	3 x 20 brisk pace	15 seconds
Leg Exchange / 15	3 x 6 moderate pace	3 x 15 brisk pace	15 seconds
Arm Swing Chest Lift / 41	2 x 20		15 seconds
Roll Up and Tuck / 23	3 x 8 moderate pace	3 x 20 brisk pace	15 seconds
Chair Push-Up / 33	3 x 4 moderate pace	3 x 12 brisk pace	15 seconds
Half Squat / 7	3 x 6 moderate pace	3 x 20 brisk pace	15 seconds
Additional exercises of your choice			
Cool Off			
Rag Doll Jog / 1	1 minute	4 minutes	
Arms Out, Up and Relax / 61	10 reps		
Over Toe Reach / 45	8 x 5 seconds		
Bent Over Sag Rotate / 49	6 x 10 seconds		

PHASE 3

EXERCISE	START AT		BUILD TO		REST BETWEEN SETS
Warm Up					
Rag Doll Jog / 1	Jog 30 seconds, walk 5 seconds, repeat 3 times		x 6		Walk 5 seconds
Lateral Side Bend / 48	2 x 15 easy rhythm				15 seconds
All Over Stretch / 56	6 reps				
Bent Over Sag / 44	6 reps				
Circuit					
Knee Push-Up / 31	10 reps		20 reps		
Half Squat / 7	10 reps		20 reps		
Bent Knee Sit Up / 22	10 reps	x 2	20 reps	x 2	
Arm Drill / 19	10 reps		20 reps		
Leg Exchange / 15	10 reps		20 reps		
Roll Up and Tuck / 23	10 reps		20 reps		
*Additional exercises of your choice					
Cool Off					
Rag Doll Jog / 1	Jog 30 seconds, walk 5 seconds, repeat 3 times		x 6		
High Stretch and Relax / 40	6 x 3 seconds				
Over Toe Reach / 45	8 x 5 seconds				
Monkey Slump / 64	6 reps				

Phase 3

This phase uses a circuit system of training which starts with a warm up, moves around a circuit of exercises for a specific number of "trips", and finishes with cooling-off movements. Heretofore, you were finished with an exercise when you had completed a certain number of sets or repetitions. In the circuit system, do each exercise in sequence 10 times, then repeat the whole series twice more.

You're at a stage in your fitness campaign when you have to do a fairly large number of repetitions of each drill. Doing these repetitions all at once can be boring. The circuit system provides variety.

Even more important, it enables you to work the cardiorespiratory system with greater intensity without creating localized muscle fatigue.

Start by doing your exercises at a moderate pace. As your condition improves, increase your speed. Keep track of how fast you can complete the circuit. When you reach what you consider your full speed for the circuit, add two repetitions to each exercise every fourth workout until you are doing each exercise 20 times in every trip through the circuit.

Do the warm-up and cool-off exercises only at the beginning and end of the circuit training – do not do them each time you go around.

If you're getting on a bit in years and are simply seeking a reasonable degree of fitness, level off once you can maintain a moderate pace. "Sprinting" around the circuit may be stressful and cause problems with tendons and ligaments that aren't quite as elastic as they once were.

CREATING YOUR OWN PROGRAM

Now you're ready for your own program. If you can handle Phase 3 at a brisk pace without excessive effort, you're in pretty good shape. Retesting has indicated the areas in which you are making progress and those in which you are not, so you should have a pretty good idea of where you need development, and where "maintenance" work will suffice.

As a matter of fact, you don't *need* to progress much further than you have right now, if you don't want to. You're at a pretty good level of fitness, and a couple of circuits around Phase 3, two or three times a week will keep you there. One workout a week will probably be sufficient if you're involved in some other form of regular physical activity. As a matter of fact, if you're jogging, swimming, cycling, skipping, dancing, playing tennis or involved in some other physical project which boosts your heart rate to your projected maximum and starts you perspiring, and you're doing it three or four times a week (weekend athletes don't qualify), you can consider dropping your exercise workout altogether (probably with the exception of flexibility and relaxation drills). But remember this: there are very few "complete" activities. Jogging's great for heart-wind-leg development, but doesn't do much for flexibility or upper-body strength. Fitness for swimming may be hard to translate into fitness for skiing or some other land-based activity.

So it's probably best not to abandon your calisthenics program altogether. See what retesting tells you after a month or so of involvement in your particular event, and let that be your guide. The intensity with which you participate and the enjoyment you feel may help to develop condition faster than a program of exercises which don't keep up your interest.

Keep this in mind when you're making a decision on the route you will travel to physical fitness: part of the joy of living is achievement. The fitter you get, the more you'll get out of all your activities, whether they be cross-country skiing, hiking, swimming, tennis, or putting in a new garden.

How Much Should You Do?

The answer to this question depends on what you are *trying* to do. Are you seeking total fitness, or do you just want to improve your cardiovascular efficiency without bothering about strength or flexibility? Are you planning to get back in shape to play a competitive sport such as tennis? Or do you want to firm up a flabby figure and use a fitness campaign as an adjunct to your diet? How much time do you have available? All these factors will affect how often you work out, how long you work out and the type of workout you do. A person in very poor condition, for example, might find that a few minutes each day is enough at the start. Later, when he or she is fairly well-conditioned, 45 minutes at least three times a week might be necessary if improvement is to continue. Once a maintenance level has been reached, three 30-minute workouts should suffice.

For general fitness, the three most important considerations are intensity, duration, and frequency.

Intensity is particularly important in upgrading the efficiency of your heart and lungs. The pulse rate during exercise is a measure of intensity and tells you how much of a training effect you are achieving. This rate will be modified by your age, sex, and state of fitness. Older persons and those in exceptionally poor condition can achieve results at a lower level.

Exercise must be vigorous enough to increase your heart rate to between 70 and 85 per cent of its maximum for a good training effect to take place. Maximum heart rate decreases with age, and a 50-year-old might have a max some 20 beats lower than when he or she was 30. This is why you usually have to cut back on your exercise intensity as you get older.

Calculate your predicted maximum heart rate by subtracting your age from 220. The resulting figure should be accurate within 10 beats. Women should add 5 to this figure.

The following table will enable you to calculate the heart rate you should seek during your workout in order to achieve a positive training effect on your heart and circulatory system, relative to your age. If you are extremely unfit, you would be wise to begin below the starting range. As your conditioning improves, strive for the target heart rate. Do not exceed the Heart Rate Limit given in the right-hand column.

If you have a history of heart disease or cardiovascular disorder, consult a physician for a Target Heart Rate more directly related to your level of restriction.

HEART-RATED EXERCISE

AGE	STARTING RANGE 70% of Max.	TARGET HEART RATE 80% of Max.	HEART RATE LIMIT 85% of Max.
Under 18	141	162	172
19 – 24	137–141	157–161	167–171
25 – 29	134–137	153–156	162–166
30 – 34	130–133	149–152	158–162
35 – 39	127–132	145–148	154–157
40 – 44	123–126	141–144	150–153
45 – 49	120–123	137–140	145–149
50 – 54	116–119	133–136	141–145
55 – 59	113–116	129–132	137-140
60 – 64	109–112	125–128	133–136
65 – 69	106–108	121–124	128–132
70 and over	105	120	128

Duration The target rate should not only be achieved, but should be sustained for a period of time. Most authorities believe that a total of 15 minutes three times a week is the *minimum* required to develop and maintain adequate levels of heart-lung fitness.

Obviously, if you are seeking high levels of fitness, the duration and frequency of your workouts should be increased.

The workout period need not be continuous, however; for example, you could achieve virtually the same effect as a steady half-hour jog at 150 beats per minute by working at this heart rate in three 10-minute periods, with brief rest intervals between.

Distance runners use this principle in their interval training. It enables them to pile on far more work than they would be able to do if they were running at a steady speed. For example, by using intervals, they can work at near maximum heart rates for long periods of time. The brief rests help to postpone exhaustion.

This is a good point to remember if your lack of fitness prevents you from maintaining an activity such as jogging, cycling, or swimming for very long at one time. Use the interval system. Jog-walk-jog-walk until you've put in a total of at least 15 minutes of jogging. Gradually you'll be able to increase the length of the jog and shorten the length of the walk until you're jogging for the whole period.

Some researchers suggest that the heart rate should be boosted past the 85 per cent mark. However, this ignores a risk factor present for older persons or those who are extremely unfit. The "Guidelines for Graded Exercise Testing and Exercise Prescription" issued by the American College of Sports Medicine suggests 20 to 30 minutes at 60 to 70 per cent of maximum for the first weeks of training when the individual is unfit, changing to 15 minutes at 70 to 85 per cent as condition improves.

The ACSM also recommends that the total workout last from 20 to 45 minutes, including warm up, cool off and exercises for areas other than the cardiovascular system.

Frequency Maximum benefits from a training session seem to last only 48 hours. This means you should plan to work out at least every other day.

Research indicates that good progress can be made with just three workouts a week, while the optimum is five. Some individuals thrive on a seven-days-a-week regime, but Dr. Jack Wilmore of the University of California believes that these persons probably have a basic psychological need to exercise without fail. Their motivation is so strong that they feel guilty when they do not work out. However, the additional physiological benefits they receive do not match the tremendous amount of time and energy expended. When planning your program remember that the body seems to demand periods of rest and replenishment.

Two workouts a week produce extremely slow progress. One workout a week does very little, and if the workout is severe it could have adverse effects, particularly for older people.

Overweight individuals who are exercising to lose pounds should keep in mind the following: An hour of vigorous exercise done three times a week might burn up 1200 calories. By exercising at higher intensity for shorter periods – say 35 minutes five times a week – you could easily boost this to 1500 calories; so if weight loss is your objective you're better off using frequent short workouts at higher intensity.

How to Progress

One of the questions that may occur to you when you are developing your exercise program is how you should progress. At what point in the number of repetitions of an exercise does the law of diminishing returns take over? Should you do 3, 6, 12 or 15 sets of 3, 6, 12 or 15 repetitions?

THE LAW OF REPETITIONS

How many times should you repeat a particular exercise for maximum benefit? It depends on what you are seeking.

If your goal is muscle endurance, the law of repetitions indicates that you should do a high number of repetitions at a brisk speed against light resistance. If it's pure strength you want, then few repetitions at a slow pace using maximum resistance (weight) is the correct method.

In fact, the law of repetitions is not really a law at all. It implies, for example, that a distance runner should sprint all out a number of times in order to develop endurance; but the body doesn't work that way. For one thing, the act of sprinting places considerable load (resistance) on certain muscles, so the runner is not adhering strictly to the law. Sprinting also cuts down the total amount of work (number of repetitions) that can be done before exhaustion sets in, so the law is disobeyed on another count. Similarly, a single maximum effort may not be the best way to develop maximum strength. It may increase the size of the muscle fibers (causing the muscle to increase in size), but it will not increase capillarization of the muscles (blood flow) which is also a factor in the expression of useful strength.

There is conflict among the researchers themselves as to the exact effects of the various methods of training. It is only in the last 20 years that intensive study of this basic human capability has been undertaken in the laboratories, and new and fascinating facts are emerging every day.

For example, the Russians and other east Europeans have found that it is possible to produce strength without exercising. They have developed a system of forcing the muscles to contract by using electric shocks. It works, and it saves time and effort, but at first glance sounds rather horrifying – although the athletes upon whom they use it apparently don't mind.

For the average person interested in overall physical fitness, the extremes of the law of repetitions are pointless. The exercises in this book have been designed to cater to an average need. Some are specifically for building strength and involve extra resistance through the use of opposing muscle groups or weights or some other device such as a rubber tension band. Still other exercises are aimed at flexibility or relaxation, and do not involve either strength or endurance.

If you find that you are doing 3 sets of 20 repetitions of any exercise at a brisk pace without undue difficulty, there probably is not much point in adding further sets or repetitions unless the instructions for that particular exercise tell you to do so. You should either increase the difficulty by adding resistance (weights, or by pressing harder when using opposing muscle groups), or find a more difficult exercise. For example, if you can do 3 sets of 20 push-ups at a brisk pace without too much rest in between, you have excellent muscle endurance in the arms, shoulders, and upper back. Make the push-ups harder by lowering yourself between 2 chairs, or by strapping a 5 lb. weight on your back. (Remember, of course, to decrease the number of repetitions and build gradually again.)

The principle of adding weight is known as progressive resistance, and is probably the simplest and most effective way for the average person to build strength and endurance at the same time. Most (although not all) exercises lend themselves to this sort of development. It may take a little ingenuity on your part to figure out exactly how, particularly if you do not want to invest in a set of weights. Books and other heavy objects held in the hand or strapped to the leg or shoes can be very useful, particularly in exercises involving jumping or lifting arms or legs. The exact amount of weight doesn't matter, although you should keep track of it on the bathroom scales so that you can measure progress.

How fast do you lose strength when you stop training? The rate of loss depends on the speed with which you acquired strength. In general, it disappears one third as fast as it was achieved. Strength gained slowly, therefore, disappears slowly, and a small amount may be retained indefinitely. One strength-training session every two weeks is sufficient to maintain it, while one every six weeks will retard strength loss considerably.

Muscular strength is defined in the *Encyclopedia of Sport Sciences and Medicine* as "the maximum force that can be exerted by a muscle on one contraction". Muscular endurance is measured in terms of "repeated contractions of a muscle working against moderate resistance".[1]

Strength and endurance are directly linked. Obviously, if we had no strength (an impossibility), we could have no endurance; similarly, strength without endurance would be useless. One big effort and we'd be finished. How much of each one do we require? – as much as we have the time and inspiration to seek out.

If you are strong but lack endurance, you should exercise in a way that emphasizes endurance. If you are weak, chances are that you lack strength *and* endurance, and should try to develop both. Strength increases endurance (within certain limitations) by making it easier for the body to move against resistance. The less effort required, the longer you can produce that effort.

Obviously, there are limits. No distance runner wants a weightlifter's build. The sheer effort of shifting all that muscle bulk would tire him or her out. There's a law of diminishing returns which cannot be ignored.

SOME FACTS ABOUT STRENGTH

Several things happen to muscles when they gain in strength (some aspects were discussed in Chapter 2, page 25). There is an increase in: 1. size of muscle fibers 2. proportion of active fibers (Research has indicated that some new fibers are created by training, but this has not yet been substantiated.), 3. protein content, 4. fluid content, 5. number of capillaries, 6. connective tissue. These changes contribute to an increase in muscle size, known as hypertrophy.

There is a decrease in: 1. fat within the muscle tissue, 2. inhibitory control of muscles (the signal which ends the muscle contraction).

Certain additional chemical changes, too complex to discuss here, also take place.

Several training methods can be used to increase strength. Knowing the meaning of some of the rather mysterious labels one hears – isometrics, isotonics, auxotonics – may help you to understand the purpose of the exercises in this book.

All the exercises in Chapter 5, for example, are isotonic, which means that they involve movement. Some of them are resistance exercises because they use weights or some other method of increasing the force against which your muscles must work, and some of them are isokinetic because near-maximum resistance is applied throughout the full range of the muscles' movement.

The following brief definitions should help to clarify what you are doing with your body during your fitness program.

Isotonic Exercise: This refers to any exercise which involves movement, as opposed to isometric exercise in which there is no movement.

Resistance Exercise: This form of exercise requires that some external resistance be opposed to the movement. Weight training is the best known form, but resistance can also be provided by a wall, or your own muscles, as when you push with one hand while resisting with the other.

Here are some principles of weight training:

1. Resistance exercises should always be done progressively, that is, with gradual increases in resistance over a period of time; otherwise there will be no increase in strength.

2. The muscles being exercised should be contracted and extended through their full range of motion. For example, when curling a barbell, start with the arms fully extended and bring the barbell all the way to the chest so the muscles are fully contracted. Increase the effectiveness of the exercise by lowering the barbell to the starting position instead of simply relaxing and letting it fall back.

3. Exercise both the agonist and antagonist muscles. For example, curling a barbell will develop the biceps but the antagonists – the triceps – will remain undeveloped. Pullovers (lifting the barbell from behind the head while in a lying-down position) will be required. Failure to do this may result in arms which remain partially flexed at the elbows because of powerful flexors and weak extensors.

4. Include stretching exercises for the joints to increase flexibility. Isometric exercises tend to increase inflexibility.

5. When developing strength for a particular sport, try to make some of the exercises as specific as possible – swimming movements for swimming, shooting movements with the arms and wrists for hockey, and so on.

6. Do not use heavy resistance exercises if you have high blood pressure.

Eccentric and Concentric Exercise: Loading the muscles when they are lengthening is eccentric exercise. Its opposite – loading the muscles when they are shortening – is concentric exercise. Most body movements involve a little of both; certain muscles are shortened, while the opposing (antagonistic) muscles lengthen, and vice versa.

The weakness of certain exercise

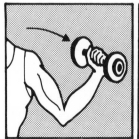 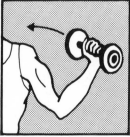

Eccentric Exercise   Concentric Exercise

movements is that they exert a training load (resistance) in only one direction. In effect, they are incomplete. Take as an example curling a barbell—lifting it in front of you by bending the arms. In this case, most of the work is done by the shortening of the biceps and certain other muscles of the arms and shoulders. This is concentric work. But if the barbell is simply dropped to the starting position again, part of the benefit is lost. By lowering it *slowly* so that the muscles are also stressed while they are lengthening, it is possible to increase the training benefits.

Apply the same principle to push-ups, sit ups, knee bends and many other exercises: return slowly to the starting position so that certain muscles are loaded while they are stretching rather than contracting. You can probably figure out eccentric phases for a number of the exercises you do; many of them already have this component built in.

The greater the variety of challenges the muscles are given, the more efficient they are likely to be in different movements demanding strength. In addition, since they will have been heavily stressed during the lengthening phase of movement they will be more injury-resistant. The skier who falls, for example, may have his limbs thrown into sudden extension, forcibly lengthening the muscles.

Isometric Exercise: In isometric exercises there is no movement. The basic objective is to meet the immovable object with irresistible force. An isometric exercise could involve, for example, pressing the palms of the hands together in front of you as hard as possible for a period of time. This movement would strengthen muscles in the chest and arms. Properly used, isometrics develop strength very fast. Unfortunately, it is strength which is fully useful only in very limited ways, since the muscle has been developed statically at a particular angle.

According to Hettinger and Muller, the German researchers who first popularized isometrics in scientific form in the 1950s (Charles Atlas and others were using it much earlier), tension held at 66 per cent of maximum for six seconds once per day will build both bulk and strength. The problem: this strength will be most useful for keeping your palms stuck together if someone wants to pull them apart. If you wanted full strength through a full range of movement, you would have to repeat this exercise for each degree of movement required.

Isometrics can be extremely useful when there is weakness at a particular point in the required action, or when an injured joint (such as a knee) requires muscles which will hold it firmly in place. It may also be effective where a large initial effort is required to overcome inertia or some other force, as in shot putting. Isometrics enables you to bulk up a specific muscle group—the pectorals, biceps, or quadriceps—if looking impressive on the beach is your objective.

For the average person, however, other forms of progressive isotonic exercise appear preferable, particularly if muscle endurance is required.

Isokinetic Exercise: This form of exercise involves keeping maximum or near-maximum resistance or load on a particular muscle group through a full range of movement. (In isometrics the muscles remain static while they are loaded.)

For an example of an isokinetic exercise, make a fist with one hand and use the palm of the other hand to push it across the chest while resisting as strongly as possible with the fist. Then push back with the fist, resisting with the palm. The amount of resistance changes throughout the movement, but remains maximal at any given time.

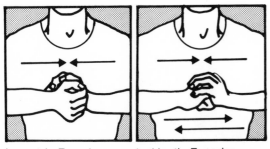

Isometric Exercise   Isokinetic Exercise

Isokinetics have certain advantages over isometrics, which develop only static strength, and over isotonic weight training in which, during much of the movement, muscles will be under less than maximum load. It is difficult to achieve maximum loading in isotonics because the muscles are limited by the amount of weight which they can handle at their *weakest* point. To understand this principle, you must remember that the limbs of the body are levers, hinged at the joints. A pull at right angles to a lever gives maximum mechanical efficiency. But when you straighten your arm, as in lifting a weight, you are wasting much of your initial strength by pulling the radius and ulna (forearm) against the humerus (upper arm). This would be the muscles' weakest point. The other would be when the arm is fully bent and the muscle can contract no further.

Isokinetics permit isotonic strength training in movements which are specific to the sports or events in which they are to be used. The drawback is that special equipment often is required to duplicate these movements.

Some experts feel that isokinetics are a step to a system of exercise known as auxotonic in which not only are the tension and length of the muscles changed throughout the movement, but also the speed of movement is changed.

Flexibility

Apart from the way loss of flexibility makes you feel, it deprives your body of one of its most important protective functions: the ability to bend and rotate through a full range of movement. When flexibility is limited, the body becomes more vulnerable to injury, particularly muscle and ligament strains or tears. This is especially true for anyone involved in sports.

There are two types of flexibility: extant and dynamic. The former is the ability to stretch the body freely in a particular direction as, for example, bending over to tie your shoes. The latter involves the capacity to twist and turn in various directions at varying speeds, as you would when climbing a tree or playing tennis.

Like so many physical capabilities, flexibility appears to be specific. You may be flexible in the shoulders but not in the back thighs, flexible in the thighs but not in the ankles. It relates partially to your physique and partially to your life style. People who sit at a desk all day, for example, may gradually lose flexibility in their hamstrings and hips because the associated muscles and ligaments lose their elasticity. Active individuals usually retain considerable flexibility.

It is the muscles' inability to stretch which causes loss of flexibility rather than an actual shortening of the muscle fibers. Conversely, increases in flexibility are created by increasing the relaxation capability of the fibers rather than by making them permanently longer.

This is one reason why it is generally considered better to do flexibility (stretching) exercises slowly rather than quickly, rhythmically rather than abruptly. There is controversy on this point, but contemporary thinking favors slow stretching and when possible holding the maximum stretch for several seconds or longer to promote the relaxation reflex of the muscles.

Quick, bouncy stretching movements can in some circumstances cause the opposite effect to the one desired. The muscle may react by going into spasm, as the patella ligament in your knee does when the doctor hits it with his little hammer. It is this spasm – known as the myotatic reflex – which causes the leg to jerk.

In addition, fast, hard, stretching movements, known as ballistic stretching, may cause injury. If your muscles and ligaments are weak and your joints inflexible, it is not difficult to overdo a movement and suffer a strain or a tear.

Fortunately, lost flexibility is fairly easily recovered. Regular stretching movements in which the muscles are progressively lengthened and the joints are flexed and/or rotated through a full range of movement (perhaps to musical accompaniment) should be included in your program.

Phase 4

In selecting your exercises for Phase 4, the following guidelines will help you create a balanced program. This program is only a sample which will be modified by your testing.

1. WARM UP

This should include some mild cardiovascular stimulation, (such as slow jogging, skipping, fast walking), one general relaxation exercise, and a couple of flexibility exercises which focus on the problem areas as revealed by testing.

2. BODY OF PROGRAM

If you are continuing with calisthenics, your program should include the following:

1. Abdominal work

2. Arms (cardiovascular exercise such as push-ups and fast arm swinging, or strength work).

3. A figure-fault exercise for your particular problems. This might mean low back/abdominal work, or an exercise to correct your tendency to slump.

4. Cardiovascular activity involving the legs (jogging, box stepping).

5. A general relaxation exercise.

6. More arm work (general or cardiovascular, depending on your needs).

7. Another abdominal exercise.

8. A figure-fault exercise of your choice, or strength work.

9. Leg work (cardiovascular).

10. A general relaxation exercise.

If your program is largely outdoor cardiovascular work (such as a half hour of jogging, swimming, or cycling), move straight from the warm up into exercises for your specific problem areas. Then do your cardiovascular work, winding up with some cool-off exercises and a shower.

3. COOL OFF

Always finish your workout with a brief session of mild activity to help the body adjust to cessation of effort so that it returns to normal in gentle stages. This should include some mild cardiovascular activity at a decreasing rate, such as relaxed jogging gradually slowing down to a walk, a flexibility exercise or two, and a general relaxation exercise.

There are several reasons why a cool-off period is necessary, the most important being to help the return flow of blood to the heart from the muscles. During exercise, the veins in the muscles become heavily loaded with blood. If you stop suddenly, the blood tends to "pool" in the veins. The lactic acid caused by your activity may not be completely removed, causing muscular stiffness and soreness later on, and, in addition, the heart may tend to beat unevenly as it struggles to get the blood flow back to normal. This is known as "arrhythmias".

Here are some general points to keep in mind.

1. Your new program may make you stiff at first. This doesn't mean that you're in worse condition than you thought. All conditioning is specific to the type of activity, and any change may affect the muscles. The stiffness will soon pass.

2. Until you reach a reasonable level of conditioning, do not program a lying-down activity immediately after a heavy cardiovascular or strength exercise. Changes in blood pressure and blood flow resulting from the sudden change in position may cause dizziness or nausea.

3. Whereas Phase 3 required doing circuits, for the first few sessions in Phase 4, move back to interval work (3 sets of 6 to 12 repetitions, for example). Every other workout add a couple of reps, and once you are

handling the program easily, move to the circuit system.

4. Start your new program fairly slowly, gradually building up the speed of movement until you achieve a good brisk pace. Stretching (flexibility) and relaxation drills are to be done slowly, of course, unless otherwise specified. Relax completely during rest intervals.

5. Your exercise program must be individual and please you. But remember this: exercises you find difficult are probably the very ones you need. The difficulty may indicate a physical shortcoming that requires attention. Don't duck the hard ones.

6. Change your exercises from time to time. Doing the same arm drills or the old familiar stretching routines week after week can be monotonous. There are many alternative exercises for each area of the body. Moreover, each exercise utilizes slightly different muscles in slightly different ways, so you get extra benefits.

5

Your
Exercise Bank

THE EXERCISES

All the exercises you need for a good basic fitness program are contained in this chapter. Every important area of the body is covered, from the feet, legs, arms, chest, abdomen and back to the cardiovascular system.

Following each exercise description there is a statement of its purpose. You may assume that those exercises which tax the respiratory response will improve cardiorespiratory efficiency.

In most cases, alternative exercises have been provided which do similar jobs, as well as variations on exercises. Variety is the key to avoiding the boredom that often results from doing the same thing over and over again, day in and day out. These alternatives and variations also use the muscles in slightly different ways; so, if one is not working to your satisfaction, try another one designed to accomplish the same ends. For you, it may be more effective.

The starting number of repetitions and the target number have been indicated after each exercise. As condition develops, add a couple of repetitions after 2 or 3 workouts until the target has been achieved. (In some instances, depending on your goal, you may wish to exceed the target reps.) There is usually a 15-second rest between sets. Where legs and arms are alternated within a movement, left-right counts as one repetition.

For example, the instructions might read:

Reps: 3x4 to 3x14   **Rest:** 15

This means: Start with 3 sets of 4 repetitions. Build to a target of 3 sets of 14 repetitions. Rest for 15 seconds between sets.

You can, if you like, draw on exercises from other sources. Make sure, however, that they are safe for you to do. The exercises listed have been coded so that you will know which ones to avoid if you have back problems or high blood pressure, for example, or what adjustment you should use to make a particular exercise safe for you. The coding is explained in the section on Contraindications on page 70.

Certain alternative exercises, or methods of doing exercises, are included in the chapter on special problems (such as a sagging abdomen or postural defects such as lordosis or kyphosis). Include these exercises in your program if you have a particular physical defect which requires attention.

Special anti-tension drills are found in the chapter on relaxation, and a number of exercises you can do at the office or in your car are listed in Chapter 9, Fitness at Work Too.

The value of physical activities such as sports, gardening, and hiking should not be underestimated. They are a vital and complementary part of any fitness campaign, particularly for those who get bored with exercise programs.

Resistance belt Some exercises described in this book require an "accessory" if they are to be done properly – an elastic belt which provides the resistance against which the muscles must work.

A belt is easy to acquire. Ask your local garage man to cut 2 or 3 circles, 1½ inches wide, from an old inner tube, or cut them yourself with a strong pair of scissors.

These loops can be used to develop progressive resistance in certain exercises. Start with one and build to the suggested number of repetitions; then add another belt and start over.

Contraindications

Persons with back problems, high blood pressure, or knee injuries should avoid certain exercises, or do them in modified form. The following code has been used to indicate which exercises fall into this category.

Adj – B: Exercise may be done if adjustment for back is observed.

Adj – K: Exercise may be done if adjustment for knee is observed.

Adj – B/P: Exercise may be done if adjustment for high blood pressure is observed.

Con – B: Not advisable for persons with back problems.

Con – K: Not advisable for persons with knee problems.

Con – B/P: Not advisable for persons with high blood pressure.

If you have a medical problem of any kind, always get clearance from your family physician before attempting activity which may cause high stress. Four of the most common areas of difficulty are heart conditions, high blood pressure, low back pain, and knee injuries. Exercises which should not be done or which require special adjustments by individuals with these handicaps are clearly indicated in the Exercise Bank.

Once you get medical clearance for a fitness program, the following hints may help you avoid further complications.

HEART CONDITIONS

Exercise only under direct instructions from your physician. There are no exceptions to this rule. Always warm up slowly and well and increase workloads gently. Fatigue should not persist after a few minutes of rest.

Stop whenever unexpected symptoms of any kind appear, particularly if there is persistent, recurring, or increasing chest pain. Skip your exercise session if you do not feel up to par, have unaccustomed symptoms of fatigue or anxiety, unusual headaches, dizziness, or pressure in the chest.

Avoid sudden exertion, particularly that caused by lifting heavy weights, which forces you to hold your breath. Do not lift heavy weights overhead. Get up slowly from the prone position, and avoid exercises in which the head falls below the waist from an upright position.

HIGH BLOOD PRESSURE

The warnings given for heart conditions also apply here. Discuss with your doctor your desire to exercise and get fit and go over with him the type of program which you should follow.

Exercise of the right kind can be an extremely valuable ally in your campaign to get your blood pressure down to acceptable levels. It should be rhythmical exercise of relatively mild intensity to start, gradually building to higher and higher levels of activity as the weeks go by. It should be relaxing, designed to stimulate blood flow and increase the efficiency of your cardiovascular system.

Research has shown that such programs are usually extremely effective in reducing blood pressure, provided they are done regularly and at least five times per week, preferably more.

Following is a short, non-strenuous program designed to be done first thing in the morning before work, or in the evening after you get home. It will give you a general physical tune-up, and it is brief enough so that eventually you can do it twice a day, when fitness permits. It will help you move into a more general program of fitness and sports activity, if you so desire.

Do the exercises in the order suggested and observe the instructions on progression. Have your doctor check your blood pressure every six months so you can measure your progress.

If you are overweight, benefits will be much more dramatic if this program is associated with proper nutrition designed to get rid of extra fat.

1. Rag Doll Jog/1 (exercise 1 in the Exercise Bank): **Reps**: 4x15 sec. to 10x15 sec. **Rest**: 15 sec. Then 4 x 20 sec. to 10 x 20 sec. **Rest**: 15 sec.

2. Simulated Crawl/39: **Reps**: 4 x 15 to 10 x 15. **Rest**: 15 sec. Then 4 x 20 to 10 x 20. **Rest**: 15 sec.

3. Stomach Pull-In/20: **Reps**: 6 x 10 to 6 x 20. **Rest**: 10 sec.

4. Quarter Squat/2: **Reps**: 6 x 10 to 6 x 40. **Rest**: 10 sec.

5. Arm Drill/19: **Reps**: 4 x 15 to 10 x 15. **Rest**: 15 sec. Then 4 x 20 to 10 x 20. **Rest**: 15 sec.

6. Arms Out, Up and Relax/p.184 **Reps**: 6.

7. Rag Doll Jog: Repeat as No. 1, including progression.

8. Cool Off: Walk about for 5 to 10 minutes, relaxing and breathing slowly and deeply. Let your muscles go especially loose on every exhale.

LOW BACK PAIN

It has been estimated that one in every two persons in North America suffers from some form of low back pain, and that more than 80 per cent of it is muscular in origin. The root cause is lack of exercise resulting in weakness of the holding muscles of the spine and of the abdominals. This means that a fitness program is your best remedy, provided your doctor gives the green light.

Special exercises for the back are given in Chapter 6 and should be an important part of your fitness campaign. Observe the contraindications and adjustments suggested in the Exercise Bank.

There are a few additional rules you should follow: When bending over, bend at the hips and knees rather than from the waist only; carry heavy objects close to the body, never lift them above the waist and never strain to hoist bulky, awkward objects, such as furniture; avoid sudden movements, particularly those involving movement from the waist; face any object you are trying to lift; sleep on a hard mattress, or one with a board under it.

KNEE INJURIES

The knee is a particularly vulnerable joint. It must carry almost your full weight, yet has very little defence against sudden twisting movements because its capacity for rotation is very slight, or against blows from the side. Athletes frequently have a legacy of knee problems. Older persons tackling tennis, squash, and other games requiring sudden, sharp changes of direction, or taking up jogging with its resultant jarring of the knee joint, may also experience difficulties.

Severe pain, swelling, or weakness in the knees should always be treated by a doctor. If there is permanent weakness, the only solution is to strengthen the muscles above and below the joint, and for this reason leg exercises involving resistance against heavy weights (or some other device such as a rubber belt) should be done. Isometric contractions of the muscles surrounding the knee are also valuable.

Avoid: deep-knee bends, full squats, and the "duck walk" exercise, which are potentially damaging to the internal supporting structures and cartilages of the knees.

What These Exercises Do

To help you put together your own program, here is a breakdown of the various areas and parts of the body upon which exercise will have an effect. Each exercise in the "Bank" is numbered. Page numbers are given for exercises from other chapters.

CARDIOVASCULAR

Rag Doll Jog—arms, legs/1
Squats—legs/2, 3, 6, 7, 8, 11, 12.
Squat Jump—legs/13
Leg Exchange—legs/15
Step Up—legs/16
Straddle Hop Arm Lift—legs/17
Shadow Skipping—arms, legs/18
Arm Drill—arms/19
Bent Knee Sit Up—abdominals/22
Roll Up and Tuck—abdominals/23
Knee/Toe Touches—abdominals/24-28
Push-Up—arms, upper body/31-36

See also: walking, jogging, rope skipping, swimming, and other cardiovascular activities in this chapter.

FLEXIBILITY

Simulated Crawl—shoulders/39
High Stretch and Relax—chest/40
Arm Swing Chest Lift—chest/41
Knee to Chest Tuck—low back, buttocks/42
Bent Over Pull-In—back thighs, low back/43
Bent Over Sag—back thighs, low back/44
Over Toe Reach—back thighs, low back/45
Arms Up, Press Back—shoulders/46
Side Bend, Hold—waist, lateral muscles/47
Lateral Side Bend—waist, lateral muscles/48
Bent Over Sag Rotate—back thighs, low back, lateral muscles/49
Torso Twist—waist, lateral muscles/50
Willow Stretch—waist, lateral muscles/51
Shoulder Rotation—shoulders/52
Back Thigh Stretch—back thigh muscles/53
Seated Calf Stretch—calf muscles/54
Calf Stretch—calf muscles/55
Allover Stretch—front and back thigh muscles, calf muscles, shoulders/56
Bent Over Sag—low back, back thigh muscles/63
Bent Arm Elbow Rotation—shoulders, chest/59

RELAXATION CONTROL

High Stretch and Relax/40
Arm Swing Chest Lift/41
Torso Twist/50
Seated Shoulder Shrug/57
Shoulder Shrug and Relax/58
Bent Arm Elbow Rotation/59
Crucifix Collapse/60
Arms Out, Up and Relax/61
Let Go Breathing/62
Bent Over Sag/63
Monkey Slump/64

See also Chapter 8, How to Reduce Tension and Learn to Relax and Chapter 9, Fitness at Work Too.

STRENGTH DEVELOPMENT

Quarter Squats – thighs / 2-6
Half Squats—thigh, buttocks, calf
  muscles / 7-12
Bent Knee Sit Up – abdominals / 22
Roll Up and Tuck – abdominals / 23
Knee/Toe Touches – abdominals / 24-28
Slow Leg Let Down—low back, abdominals,
  shoulders, upper body / 29
Push-Ups—arms, shoulders, upper
  body / 31-36
Fist Press – arms, chest / 37
Rowing Push-Pull – arms, chest / 38

The following exercises can be found in
Chapter 6, Special Problems:

Seated Leg Extension—knees, thighs / p. 120
Cushion Squeeze Half Squat—inner
  thigh / p. 117
Seated Knee Press—inner thigh / p. 117
Standing Heel Lift—hamstrings / p. 119
Cross Leg Pull-In—hamstrings / p. 119
Toe Heel Rock—knees, calves and lower
  legs / p. 121
High Stretch Pull-In Hold—abdomen / p. 122
Seated Stomach Pull-In Hold—abdomen
  p. 123
Hip Lift —buttocks, back thigh / p. 124
Straight Leg Back Lift—buttocks, and back
  thigh / p. 124
Resisted Leg Lift—back thigh, buttocks
  p. 125
Fist Push Around—chest / p. 135
Resistance Press Down—chest / p. 136
Forward Arm Lift—shoulders / p. 137
Lateral Arm Lift—shoulders / p. 137
Arm Circles—shoulders / p. 137
Head Circling—neck / p. 138
Resistance Drill—neck / p. 138
The Bull Dog—neck, chin / p. 138
Knee Press Down—triceps / p. 139
Push-Pull—triceps / p. 139
Resisted Arm Lift—arms / p. 140
Single Arm Resistance—arms / p. 141

POSTURE DEFECTS

Lordosis
Stomach Pull-In / 20
Bent Knee Sit Up / 22
Roll Up and Tuck / 23
Inhale-Exhale / 30
Lying Knee to Chest Tuck / 42
Bent Over Sag / 44
Over Toe Reach / 45
Seated Bent Over Sag / 63
Low Back Press Down / p. 133
Supine Knee Pull / p. 134

Scoliosis
Keynote Bend / p. 132
Seated Bend Rotate / p. 130
Bar Hang / p. 130

Kyphosis
Head Pull Back Hold / p. 126
Elbows Back Hold / p. 126
Book Press / p. 128
Straight/Bent Arm Pull Back / p. 129

Shoulder Blades
Wall Press / p. 128
Bent Arm Lateral Pull Back / p. 129
Straight/Bent Arm Pull Back / p. 129

Feet
Caterpillar Crawl / 65
Arch Lift and Hold / 66
Marble Pick Up / 67
Pigeon-Toed Stepover / 68
Rock and Lift / 69
Foot Roll / 70

SEXERCISES

Seated Knee Press—inner thigh / p. 117
Hip Lift—buttocks, back thigh / p. 124
Cushion Squeeze Half Squat—inner thigh,
  front thighs / p. 117

GENERAL

See Chapter 6, Special Problems and
Chapter 9, Fitness at Work Too.

70 EXERCISES

1. RAG DOLL JOG

Jog on the spot at medium pace, lifting feet about 6 inches off the ground. Allow your muscles to go as limp and floppy as possible, particularly the hands, arms, shoulders, and neck. Try to imitate a jogging rag doll. Pretend you have no bones in your limbs at all. To aid in relaxing the upper body, rest tongue gently behind lower teeth, and keep thumb and middle finger in light contact.

> **Reps:** 30 sec. to 4 min.
>
> **Purpose:** Relaxation and cardiovascular warm up.

2. QUARTER SQUAT

Stand with arms straight out in front at about shoulder height with feet hip-width apart. Do a quarter squat by bending knees and lowering buttocks as if about to sit in an imaginary chair, but stop when you get about halfway to the chair. Keep feet flat on floor.

> **Reps:** 3x10 to 3x30   **Rest:** 15
>
> **Purpose:** Tones the thigh muscles.

3. QUARTER SQUAT KNEES FORWARD

Do a quarter squat by bending the knees and pushing them well forward. Keep feet flat on the floor and pointing straight ahead. Attempt to keep the body in a straight line between knees and shoulders, leaning back slightly to maintain balance.

> **Reps:** 3x10 to 3x30   **Rest:** 15
>
> **Purpose:** Tones the thigh muscles.

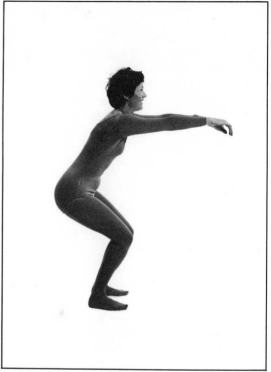

2. Quarter Squat

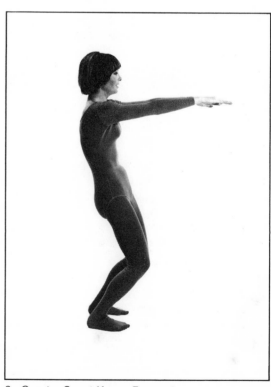

3. Quarter Squat Knees Forward

4. QUARTER SQUAT WEIGHT SHIFTED

Do a quarter squat but shift weight to the side as you go down so that you "load" one leg and then the other on alternate squats. Keep feet flat on floor and pointing straight ahead.

Reps: 3x8 to 3x30   Rest: 15

Purpose: Tones and strengthens thigh muscles.

5. SINGLE LEG QUARTER SQUAT

Holding a chair for balance, lift one leg out in front about 4 inches off the floor keeping it straight. Do a quarter squat on the other leg. Alternate legs. Eventually you should be able to discard the chair.

Con – K

Reps: 3x6 to 3x20   Rest: 15

Purpose: Tones and strengthens thigh muscles.

6. QUARTER SQUAT BOUNCE

Do a quarter squat (2) but instead of returning to starting position, bounce up and down a few inches as if your knees were shock absorbers. Keep feet flat on floor, toes pointing straight ahead.

Reps: 3x10 to 3x30   Rest: 15

Purpose: Develops tone and strengthens thigh muscles.

7. HALF SQUAT

Stand with arms straight out in front at about shoulder height, feet hip-width apart. Do a half squat by bending knees and lowering buttocks as if to sit in an imaginary chair. Keep feet flat on floor, toes pointing straight ahead.

Reps: 3x6 to 3x20   Rest: 15

Purpose: Tones thigh and calf muscles.

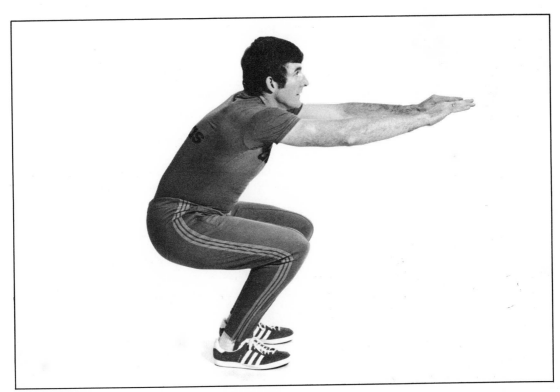

7. Half Squat

8. HALF SQUAT KNEES FORWARD

Do a half squat (7) pushing the knees well forward. Keep feet flat on the floor, toes pointed straight ahead.

Reps: 3x4 to 3x20   **Rest:** 15

Purpose: Tones thigh and calf muscles.

9. HALF SQUAT WEIGHT SHIFTED

Do a half squat (7) shifting weight to the side so that you load one leg, then the other on alternate squats.

Reps: 3x4 to 3x20   **Rest:** 15

Purpose: Tones and strengthens thigh and calf muscles.

10. SINGLE LEG HALF SQUAT

Holding a chair for balance, lift one leg out in front about 4 inches off the floor, keeping it straight. Do a half squat on the other leg. Alternate legs. Eventually eliminate chair.

Con – K

Reps: 3x2 to 3x14   **Rest:** 15

Purpose: Tones and strengthens thigh and calf muscles.

11. HALF SQUAT BOUNCE

Do a half squat (7), but instead of returning to starting position, bounce from half to quarter squat position.

Reps: 3x10 to 3x20   **Rest:** 15

Purpose: Develops strength and endurance of thigh muscles.

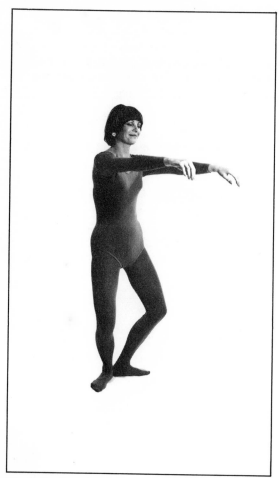

12. Ballet Squat

12. BALLET SQUAT

Do a quarter squat. Keep the heels together, with the toes and knees pointed out to the sides.

Reps: 3x8 to 3x30   **Rest:** 15

Purpose: Tones and strengthens thigh muscles.

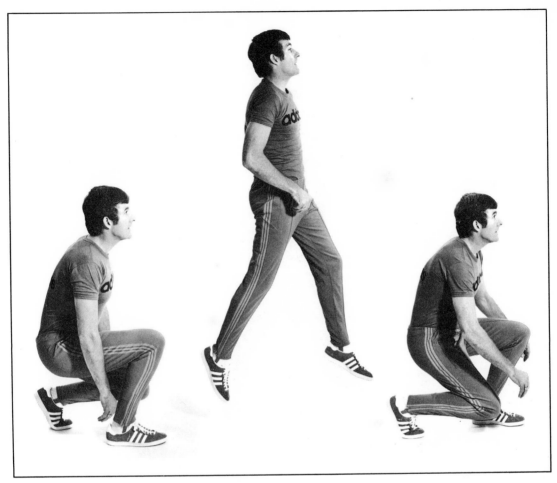

13. Squat Jump

13. SQUAT JUMP

Stand with one foot about 12 inches in front of the other. Go down to a half squat, and then jump in the air as high as you can, landing with feet reversed in the squat position. Alternate leg position each time you jump.

Reps: 3x6 to 3x14   **Rest:** 15

Purpose: Develops endurance and power in leg muscles, and cardiorespiratory efficiency.

14. FOOT VARIATIONS

Almost all the above squats can and should be done from 4 different foot positions.
1. feet flat on floor, toes pointing straight ahead
2. feet flat on floor, toes pointing out
3. on tiptoe, toes pointing straight ahead
4. on tiptoe, toes pointing out
Try these different positions on alternate days, or during alternate sets, if you prefer.

Purpose: To vary the effect on the muscle groups involved. The tiptoe position tones the calf muscles in particular.

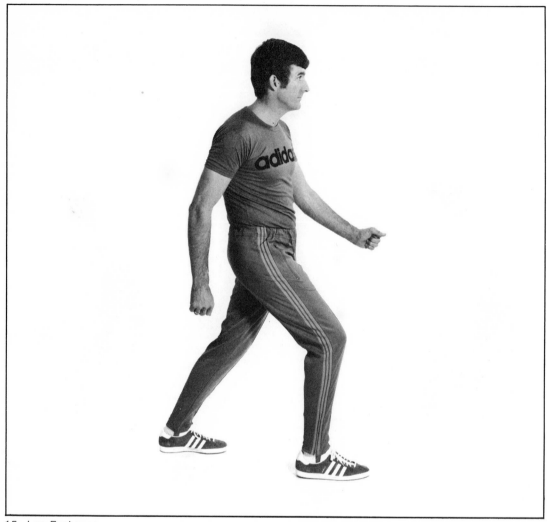

15. Leg Exchange

15. LEG EXCHANGE

Stand with one foot about 18 inches in front of the other, knees slightly bent. Now, exchange legs with a little jump. Continue at an easy pace. As you progress, increase the speed of movement and the distance between your feet.

Adj—B: Do not increase stride length.

Reps: 3x8 to 3x20   **Rest:** 15

Purpose: Increases muscle endurance of legs and cardiorespiratory efficiency.

16. STEP UP

For this exercise you'll need a strong box or stool 9 to 10 inches high. Step up on stool with right leg, bring left foot up beside it and then step down again with right. Tempo should be about one complete step up and down every 2 seconds. Change the lead leg every 5 steps.

Reps: 3x10 to 3x30   **Rest:** 15

Purpose: Improves muscle endurance of legs and cardiovascular efficiency.

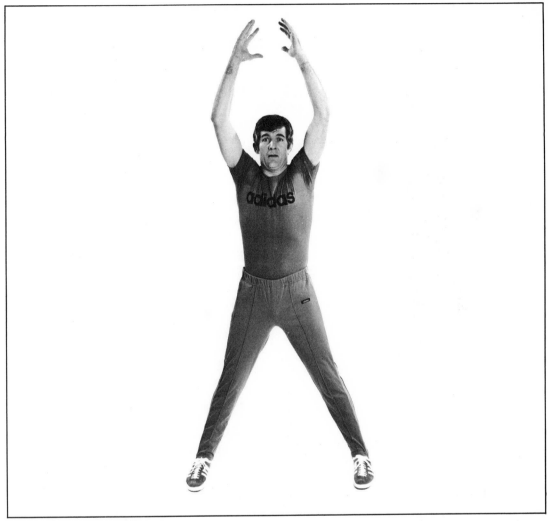

17. Straddle Hop Arm Lift

17. STRADDLE HOP ARM LIFT

Stand with feet together, toes pointing straight ahead, arms at sides. Do a straddle jump, spreading your feet about 18 inches apart, swinging your arms out to the sides, and then clapping your hands together overhead. Gradually widen straddle. Use knees as shock absorbers when landing.

Adj – B: Do not widen straddle.

Reps: 3x8 to 3x30   **Rest:** 15

Purpose: Conditions the cardiovascular system and tones the inner thigh.

18. SHADOW SKIPPING

Pretend you are skipping rope, landing with both feet. The body should stay loose and relaxed. As your condition improves, increase your skipping speed and bounce higher to increase the vigor of the drill. Use knees as shock absorbers when landing.

Adj—B: Stagger feet slightly

Reps: 1 minute to 4 minutes

Purpose: Conditions the cardiovascular system and tones leg muscles.

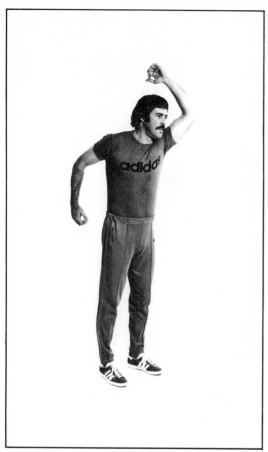

19. Arm Drill

19. ARM DRILL

Stand comfortably, feet hip-width apart.
Swing arms in an exaggerated running action,
lifting hands fairly high in front and swinging
well back. Jaw and shoulders should be loose
and relaxed.

>   **Adj – B:** Stagger feet slightly

>   **Reps:** 3x12 to 3x30   **Rest:** 15

>   **Purpose:** Conditions the cardiovascular
>   system and tones arm muscles.

20. STOMACH PULL-IN

Sit erect on a chair. While exhaling, pull
stomach in and up as far as possible. Keep
the jaw and upper body loose. Relax and
inhale. Repeat rhythmically about once every
2 seconds. If you get dizzy, breathe in a less
exaggerated manner.

>   **Reps:** 3x8 to 3x20   **Rest:** 15

>   **Purpose:** Tones abdominal muscles.

21. STOMACH PUMPING

Sit on the front edge of a chair with your
body erect, hands on knees and feet flat on
floor. Pull your stomach in as far as you can,
then let it relax and bulge outward. Breathe
rhythmically as you continue this action at a
moderately fast pace, exhaling as you pull the
abdomen in, inhaling as you pump out.

>   **Reps:** 3x8 to 3x20   **Rest:** 15

>   **Purpose:** Tones abdominal muscles.

22. BENT KNEE SIT-UP

Lie on your back with your knees well bent,
feet flat on floor and arms extended
overhead. Sit up quickly and reach past your
knees to touch toes. Relax and repeat. If you
can't reach toes at first, start with your knees
and work toward toes gradually. Tempo
should be moderate at first, increasing as
your condition improves. Use abdominals *not*
back muscles to sit up – curl up.

>   **Reps:** 3x4 to 3x24   **Rest:** 15

>   **Purpose:** Tones and strengthens
>   abdominal muscles.

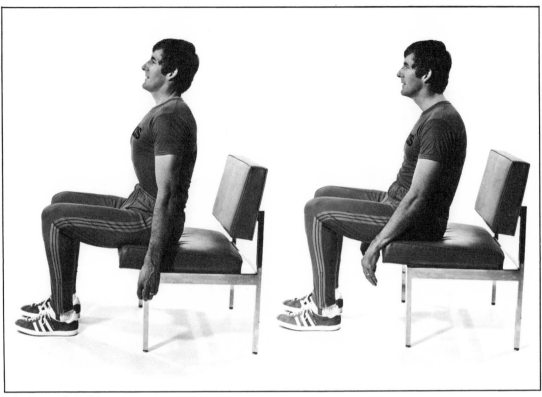

20. Stomach Pull-In

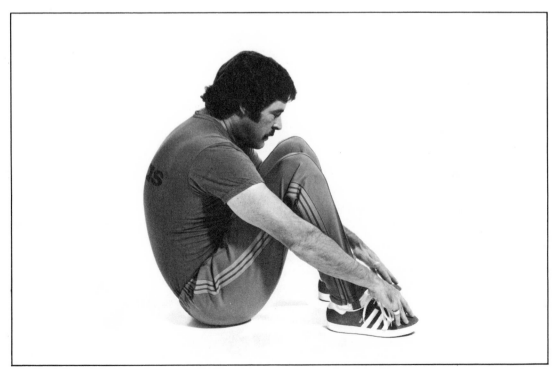

22. Bent Knee Sit-Up

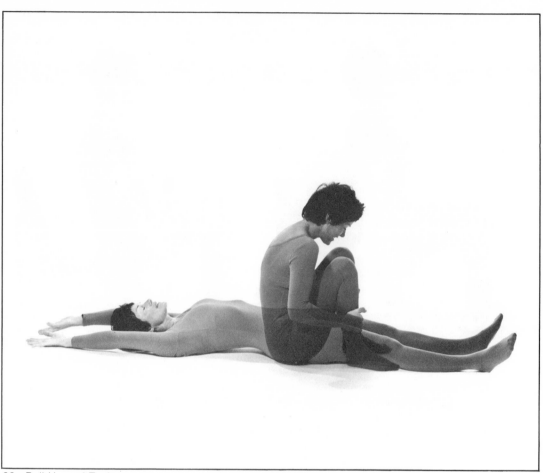

23. Roll Up and Tuck

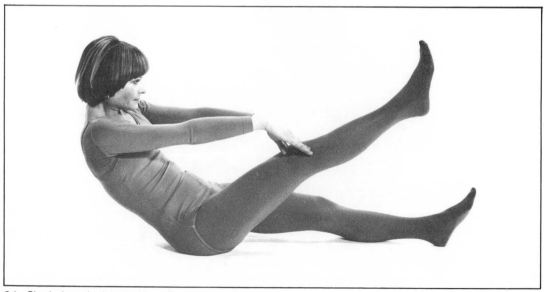

24. Single Leg Jack-knife Knee Touch

23. ROLL UP AND TUCK

Lie on your back with legs straight and arms on the floor over your head. With a quick action, curl your head and upper body forward, and simultaneously bend your knees and lift them toward your stomach so you finish in a fully tucked position, knees to chest, hands grasping ankles. Return to starting position and repeat.

Reps: 3x4 to 3x24   **Rest:** 15

Purpose: Strengthens and tones abdominal muscles.

24. SINGLE LEG JACK-KNIFE KNEE TOUCH

Lie on your back with legs straight and hands stretched out overhead. Raise the upper body and one leg simultaneously, touching the knee with the hands. Keep the leg straight. Return to starting position and repeat with other leg.

Adj—B: Bend legs slightly.

Reps: 3x4 to 3x12   **Rest:** 15

Purpose: Strengthens and tones abdominal muscles.

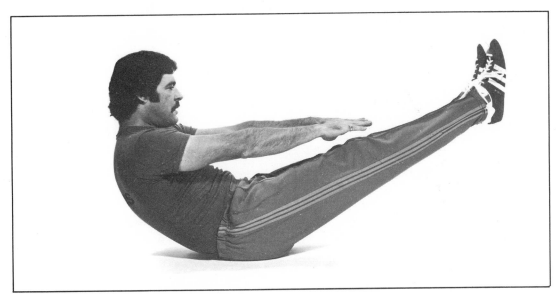

26. Double Leg Jack-knife Knee Touch

25. SINGLE LEG JACK-KNIFE

Lie on back with legs straight and hands stretched out overhead. Raise the upper body and one leg simultaneously, touching the toes with fingertips. Keep the leg straight. Return to starting position and repeat with other leg.

Adj—B: Bend legs slightly.

Reps: 3x4 to 3x12   **Rest:** 15

Purpose: Strengthens and tones abdominal muscles.

26. DOUBLE LEG JACK-KNIFE KNEE TOUCH

Follow the same procedure as for the Single Leg Jack-Knife Knee Touch but lift both legs at the same time.

Adj—B: Bend legs slightly.

Reps: 3x4 to 3x14   **Rest:** 15

Purpose: Strengthens and tones abdominal muscles.

27. DOUBLE LEG JACK-KNIFE

Follow the same procedure as for the Single Leg Jack-Knife but lift both legs simultaneously.

Adj – B: Bend legs slightly.

Reps: 3x4 to 3x14   **Rest:** 15

Purpose: Strengthens and tones abdominal muscles.

28. DOUBLE LEG JACK-KNIFE ELBOW TOUCH

Lie on back with hands clasped behind head, legs straight. Lift upper body and legs at the same time, and touch elbows to knees. Keep legs as straight as possible.

Adj – B: Bend legs slightly.

Reps: 3x4 to 3x14   **Rest:** 15

Purpose: Strengthens and tones abdominal muscles.

29. SLOW LEG LET DOWN

Lie on back with hands at sides, knees bent and feet on floor. Lift one leg until it is vertical. Slowly lower it to the floor. Alternate legs each set.

Reps: 4x6 to 4x10   **Rest:** 15

Purpose: Strengthens low back and abdominal muscles.

30. INHALE-EXHALE

Sit erect in a straight-backed chair. Inhale deeply, expanding your chest and pulling in your stomach as far as you can. Hold for 2 or 3 seconds, then exhale and pump your stomach out.

Reps: 2x5 to 2x10   **Rest:** 20

Purpose: Develops breathing response, chest expansion, and tones abdominal muscles.

31. KNEE PUSH-UP

Lie on stomach with legs bent at right angles to the floor and hands on floor directly under shoulders. Push up until arms are straight. The feet must remain over the knees and the body must be kept straight. Return to starting position slowly (don't flop).

Reps: 3x4 to 3x20   **Rest:** 15

Purpose: Strengthens and tones muscles of the arms, shoulders, and upper body.

32. STANDARD PUSH-UP

Lie on stomach with hands directly under shoulders. Push up until arms are straight. Do not drop the hips or bend at the waist. Lower body until chest barely touches the floor. Do also with variations:

Wide Push-Up: hands farther than shoulder-width apart

Narrow Push-Up: hands close together

Reps: 3x4 to 3x14   **Rest:** 15

Purpose: Strengthens and tones muscles of the arms, shoulders, and upper body.

33. CHAIR PUSH-UP

Use a sturdy arm chair, two boxes, or anything else that will provide strong support about shoulder-width apart. Place hands on supports and assume a finished push-up position. Lower body, trying to get chest down as far as possible. Keep body straight.

Reps: 3x4 to 3x14   **Rest:** 15

Purpose: Strengthens muscles of arms, shoulders, and upper body.

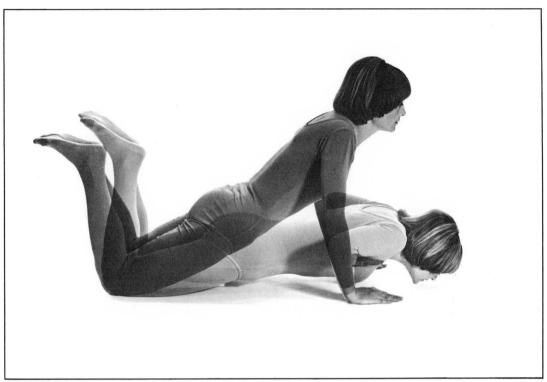

31. Knee Push-Up

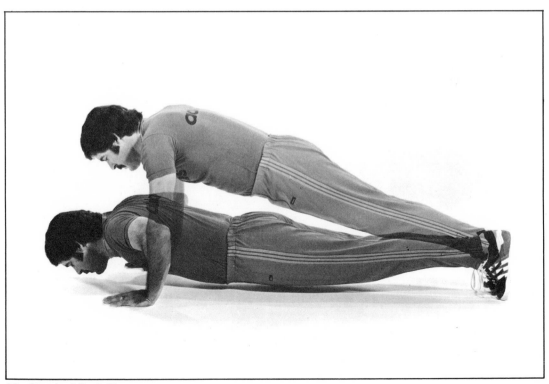

32. Standard Push-Up

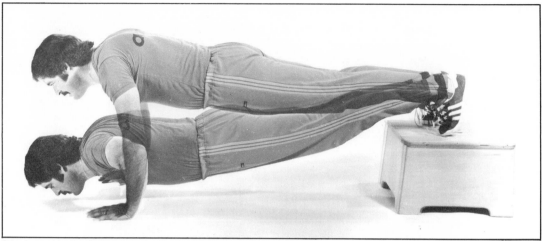

34. Legs Up Push-Up

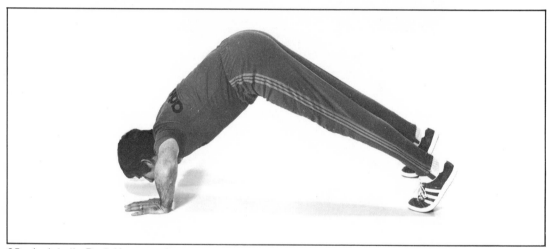

35. Jack-knife Push-Up

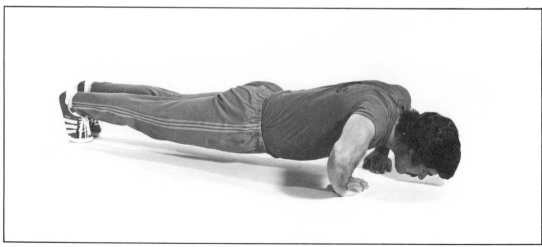

36. Inverted Push-Up

34. LEGS UP PUSH-UP

Assume finished push-up position with feet elevated on chair or box. Lower body until chest barely touches floor. Try wide and narrow hand positions. Keeps body perfectly straight.

> **Reps:** 3x4 to 3x14   **Rest:** 15
>
> **Purpose:** Strengthens muscles of arms, shoulders, and upper body.

35. JACK-KNIFE PUSH-UP

From finished push-up position, elevate buttocks so that your body forms an upside-down V. Lower the body until chin touches floor. The higher the buttocks, the more difficult the push-up. Try wide and narrow hand positions.

> **Reps:** 3x4 to 3x14   **Rest:** 15
>
> **Purpose:** Strengthens muscles of the arms, shoulders, and upper body.

36. INVERTED PUSH-UP

Do standard push-up but with hands turned so that they are pointing toward each other. Try wide and narrow hand positions. Inverted hand position can be used in all variations of push-ups.

> **Reps:** 3x4 to 3x14   **Rest:** 15
>
> **Purpose:** Strengthens muscles of the arms, shoulders, and upper body.

37. FIST PRESS-PULL

Place your left fist in front of your right fist just in front of your chin. Elbows should be in median position—about halfway to shoulder height. Press left fist out with right fist, resisting with left arm, until arms are fully extended. Then pull back to starting position, resisting with the right arm. Reverse position of your hands and repeat. Do not hold breath during this exercise.

> **Reps:** 2x4 to 2x8   **Rest:** 15
>
> **Purpose:** Strengthens muscles of the arms and upper body.

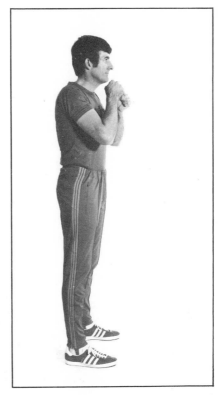

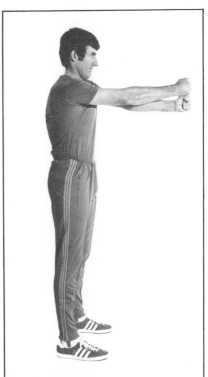

37. Fist Press-Pull

38. ROWING PUSH-PULL

Make a fist with right hand and clasp it with the other hand, palm over the top of the fist. Extend arms straight out in front at shoulder height. Pull in slowly with the left hand resisting strongly with the clenched right hand until hands are at base of neck. Now push out with right hand, resisting strongly with the left. Change hand position and repeat. Don't hold your breath.

> **Reps:** 2x4 to 2x8   **Rest:** 15

> **Purpose:** Strengthens and tones muscles of the arms and chest.

39. SIMULATED CRAWL

Stand with feet comfortably apart, and pretend you are doing the crawl swimming stroke. Carry the elbow high and get a good shoulder lift as you bring each arm forward. Swim loose and easy, keeping the jaw relaxed. Rhythm should be moderate – about one stroke per second.

> **Reps:** 2x20   **Rest:** 15

> **Purpose:** Relaxation and shoulder flexibility.

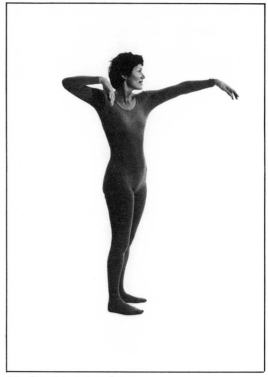

39. Simulated Crawl

40. HIGH STRETCH AND RELAX

Stand erect and stack your hands on top of your head. While taking a deep breath, reach high overhead, lifting the chest and moving the head back slightly. Stretch slowly until you've got your hands as high as they will go. Hold for 3 seconds. Now exhale, letting the air out with a long, easy sigh, while dropping your arms slowly to your sides. Let your shoulders sag, the head fall forward, and the knees go loose and slightly bent. Remain in this relaxed position for 3 to 5 seconds. Allow all the tension to seep out of the neck, arms, shoulders, and chest muscles.

> **Reps:** 6x3 sec.

> **Purpose:** Overall stretch and relaxation.

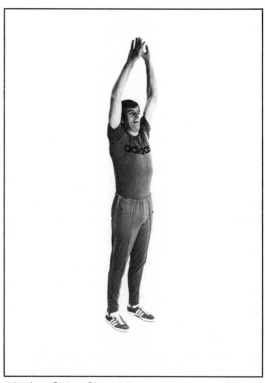

41. Arm Swing Chest Lift

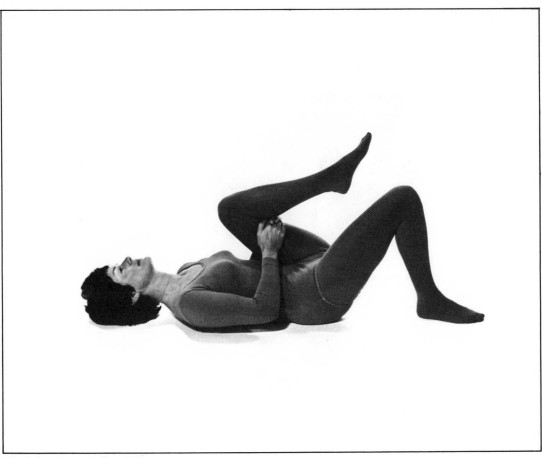

42. Lying Knee to Chest Touch

41. ARM SWING CHEST LIFT

Stand with arms at sides, feet comfortably apart. Raise both arms out to the side and up overhead, breathing in deeply at the same time. Stretch as high as you can, keeping the hands and arms relaxed while you lift the rib cage and stretch the chest region generally. Then exhale and let the arms swing back down along the same arc with the hands crossing over slightly in front of the body before you repeat the overhead lift. Keep the movement loose and rhythmic.

Reps: 2x20   **Rest:** 15

Purpose: Relaxation and stretching of chest area.

42. LYING KNEE TO CHEST TUCK

Lie on back with knees bent, feet flat on floor. Grasp behind one knee with both hands and draw it slowly up to your chest, pressing the back against the floor at the same time. Hold for a moment, lower slowly to starting position and repeat with other leg.

Reps: 3x8 to 3x14   **Rest:** 15

Purpose: Improves low back flexibility.

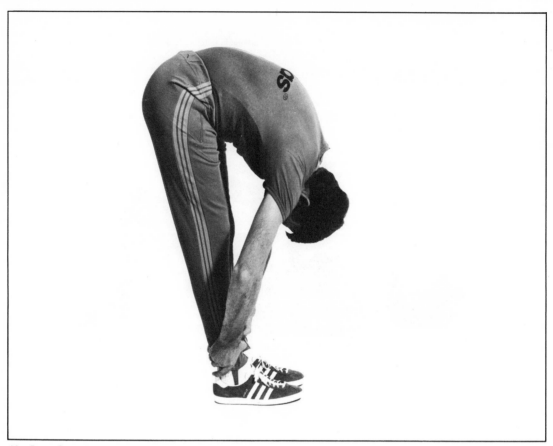

43. Bent Over Pull-In

43. BENT OVER PULL-IN

Stand erect with feet a few inches apart.
Bending from waist, slide palms down backs
of legs as low as possible. Keep knees
straight. Grasping legs, pull your chest in
against thighs. Hold for 5 seconds. Relax and
repeat. Do not hold breath.

Con – B/P

Adj – B: Bend knees slightly.

Reps: 6x5 sec.   **Rest:** 5

Purpose: Improves low back and back
thigh flexibility.

44. BENT OVER SAG

Stand with feet comfortably apart, arms
relaxed at sides. While exhaling, let the head
and upper body fall forward from the waist.
Keep the legs straight. Dangle head and arms
loosely for 3 to 5 seconds, and return slowly
to starting position as you inhale.

The forward stretch should not be forced or
exaggerated. The weight of your upper body
should exert pull on your lower back and
back thigh muscles.

Adj—B: Bend knees slightly.

Con – B/P

Reps: 6 reps.

Purpose: Relaxation, and low back and
back thigh flexibility.

45. OVER TOE REACH

Sit on floor with legs extended in front, knees straight and toes cocked back. Bend forward and reach down your legs as far as you can while exhaling. Hold maximum stretch for 5 seconds, keeping knees on floor. You may clasp your legs and pull gently to increase the stretching pressure. *Slowly* return to starting position while inhaling. Your objective is to become flexible enough to grab your insteps.

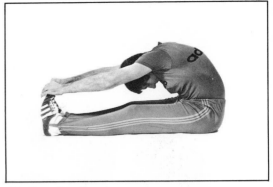

45. Over Toe Reach

Adj — B: Bend legs slightly.

Reps: 8x5 sec.

Purpose: Improves low back and back thigh flexibility.

46. ARMS UP, PRESS BACK

Stand erect, feet shoulder-width apart, arms extended downwards with palms together. Keeping arms straight, lift them overhead and back as far as you can. Press back hard for 5 seconds and return to starting position. Exhale on the upswing, inhale on the down.

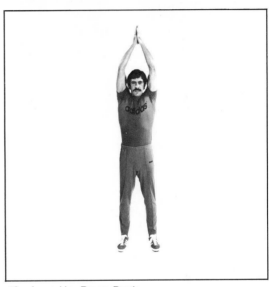

46. Arms Up, Press Back

Reps: 8x5 sec.   **Rest:** 5

Purpose: Improves tone and flexibility of shoulder area.

47. SIDE BEND, HOLD

Stand erect, arms at sides, feet comfortably apart. Move one arm down leg as far as you can, bending from the waist. Do not let hips swing out in the opposite direction. Hold maximum stretch for 5 seconds, relax and repeat to other side.

Adj — B: Do slowly and well within range of movement.

Reps: 6x5 sec. to 10x5 sec.

Purpose: Improves flexibility of muscles of the side.

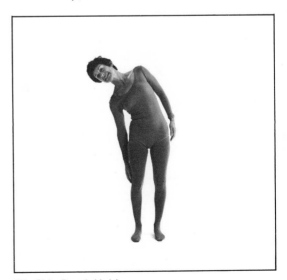

47. Side Bend, Hold

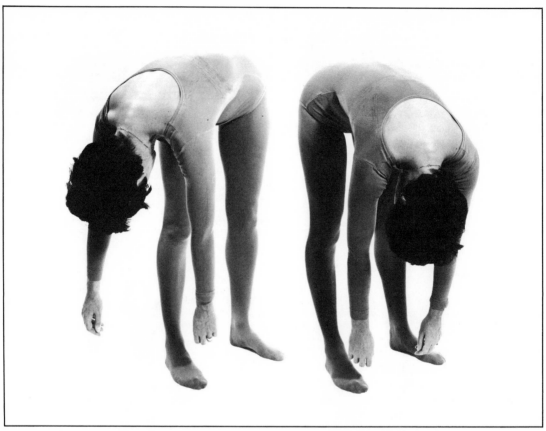

49. Bent Over Sag Rotate

48. LATERAL SIDE BEND

Stand with hands at sides, feet comfortably apart. Move one arm down leg as low as possible, bending from the waist. Do not bend forward or swing out opposite hip. Repeat rhythmically from side to side.

Adj – B: Do slowly and well within range of movement.

Reps: 2x10 to 2x20   **Rest:** 15

Purpose: Improves flexibility of muscles of the side.

49. BENT OVER SAG ROTATE

Stand erect, feet comfortably apart, head up. Let your upper body drop forward and rotate from side to side with a slight bouncing action so that you stretch the backs of your thighs and your back muscles. Make sure you keep your knees straight but allow your head to hang loosely. Let the weight of the upper body do the stretching for you—don't reach for it. Dangle loosely for 10 seconds.

Con – B/P

Adj – B: Bend knees slightly.

Reps: 6x10 sec.   **Rest:** 5

Purpose: Relaxation and flexibility of low back and back thigh muscles.

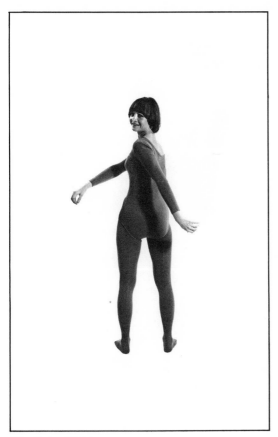

50. Torso Twist

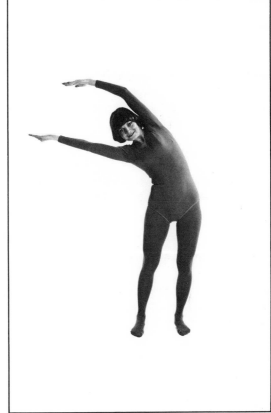

51. Willow Stretch

50. TORSO TWIST

Stand with feet comfortably apart, knees slightly bent, arms at sides. Twist your torso around to the right as far as possible, turning the head until you are looking behind you. Now twist around to the opposite side, letting the arms follow your torso around, swinging loosely with the hands and wrists relaxed. Move at a comfortable pace, twisting as far as you can without excessive muscular effort.

Reps: 2x8 to 2x14   **Rest:** 15

Purpose: Improves flexibility and tone of waist muscles.

51. WILLOW STRETCH

Stand with arms straight overhead, feet comfortably apart. Bend as far to the right as you can without forcing yourself, keeping arms close to the head. Do not bend forward or sway the hips out to the opposite side. Repeat to left.

Con—B and **B/P**

Reps: 2x4 to 2x10   **Rest:** 15

Purpose: Tones waist muscles and develops flexibility.

52. SHOULDER ROTATION

Stand with feet comfortably apart. Raise elbows sideways to shoulder height, allowing your forearms and hands to dangle loosely. Rotate elbows forward in large circles at a medium pace, keeping hands and arms loose throughout. Move the shoulders in as large an arc as possible.

   Reps: 2x20   **Rest:** 15

   Purpose: Improves shoulder flexibility and relaxation of shoulder girdle.

53. BACK THIGH STRETCH

Keeping feet flat, crouch down and place palms on floor about 2 feet in front of your toes. *Slowly* straighten your legs until knees are locked; it is important to keep head tucked into knees. If you can manage this without difficulty, bring your hands closer to your feet and try again. Find a hand position in which you can just manage to straighten the legs. Hold maximum stretch position for 5 seconds. Remember to stretch slowly.

   When your hamstrings become fully flexible, you'll be able to handle this exercise with your hands right in front of your toes.

   Con – B/P

   Reps: 6x5 sec.   **Rest:** 5

   Purpose: Improves flexibility in back thighs, hips, and lower back.

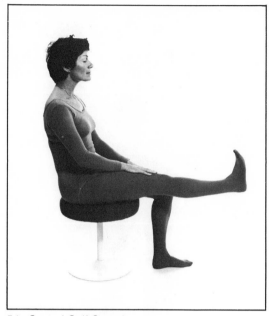

54. Seated Calf Stretch

54. SEATED CALF STRETCH

Sit erect in a chair with feet flat on floor. Lift one leg until it is horizontal to floor, reaching out with the heel and pulling toes back toward your shin as hard as you can. You should feel the stretching action in your calves and achilles tendons. Hold full stretch for 5 seconds, relax and repeat with other leg.

   Reps: 6x5 sec.

   Purpose: Improves flexibility of calf muscles.

55. CALF STRETCH

Place your hands against a wall at about shoulder height and slowly shuffle your feet away from the wall, pressing your heels against the floor as you do. When you get to maximum stretch, hold for 5 seconds.

   Reps: 8x5 sec.

   Purpose: Improves flexibility of muscles and tendons of the calves.

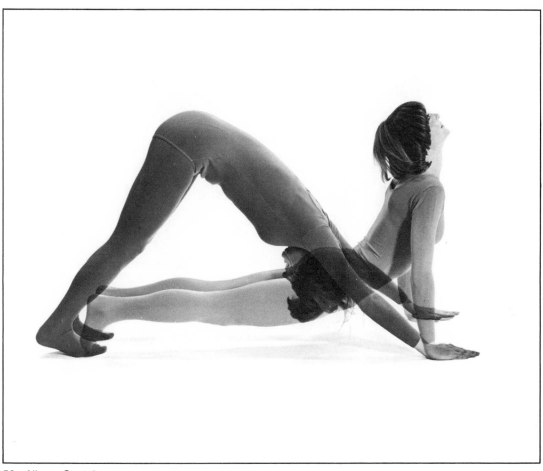

56. Allover Stretch

56. ALLOVER STRETCH

Assume the finished push-up position, hands directly under shoulders. Drop hips to floor, keeping arms straight and lifting head up and back. Hold for 3 seconds, then raise hips as high as you can, pull stomach in, and tuck head in toward chest. Hold 3 seconds, drop hips and repeat. Do not move hands or feet. Like all static stretching drills, this must be done *slowly*.

Adj – B: Avoid full arch of back in down position.

Reps: 6x3 sec.

Purpose: Improves body flexibility.

57. SHOULDER SHRUG AND RELAX

Stand with feet comfortably apart. As you take a deep breath, shrug shoulders up to ears and moderately tighten muscles throughout the body. Hold for 3 to 5 seconds. Now exhale with a long deep sigh, letting your muscles go loose so that the knees bend slightly and the head drops forward to the chest.

Reps: 6x3 sec.

Purpose: Relaxation.

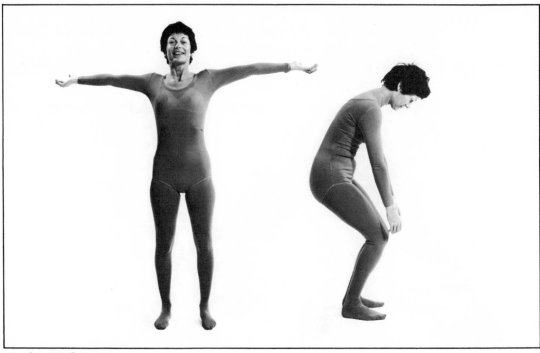

60. *Crucifix Collapse*

58. SHRUGGING

Sit with feet flat on floor. Take a deep breath and shrug the shoulders up to the ears, moderately tensing muscles throughout the body. Exhale and let shoulders drop. Repeat rhythmically.

> **Reps:** 3x10   **Rest:** 15
>
> **Purpose:** Relaxation.

59. BENT ARM ELBOW ROTATION

Stand with arms at shoulder height and bent at right angles, forearms parallel to the ground. Now force the elbows as far back as you can so you feel the pressure between your shoulder blades. Next lift elbows and shoulders upwards and rotate the arms (still bent) in large circles, first frontwards, then backwards. Alternate directions with each set.

> **Reps:** 3x10 to 3x20   **Rest:** 10
>
> **Purpose:** Relaxation and shoulder flexibility.

60. CRUCIFIX COLLAPSE

Stand with feet comfortably apart, arms out to sides at shoulder height, palms up. Take a deep breath, stiffen your whole body slightly and hold for 3 to 5 seconds. Let everything relax. Slump forward — let arms fall to sides, head and chin drop, and sag loosely at the knees.

> **Reps:** 10x3 sec.
>
> **Purpose:** Relaxation.

61. ARMS OUT, UP AND RELAX

Stand erect with feet comfortably apart. Lift arms out to sides and up overhead, simultaneously pulling stomach in and lifting chest. When you've reached as high as you can, let arms drop loosely down. Allow head to sag so chin touches chest and knees go "soft". Try to get as loose and limp as you can — feel the tension drain out.

> **Reps:** 10
>
> **Purpose:** Relaxation

62. LET GO BREATHING

Lie on back and begin to breathe slowly and deeply from the *stomach* (many people breathe shallowly from the chest only). As you inhale, let stomach puff up and as you exhale let it collapse. Repeat with a slow and easy rhythm, concentrating on allowing your whole body to go as limp and loose as possible with every exhalation. *Do not tense up first.*

Reps: 3x10   **Rest:** 15

Purpose: Relaxation.

63. SEATED BENT OVER SAG

Sit with feet shoulder-width apart, hands on knees. Take a deep breath, then exhale, allowing the upper body to fall between the legs. Now "bounce" – lift your upper body a few inches, drop it loosely, and repeat. Can also be done from a standing position with the knees bent slightly.

Reps: 10

Purpose: Relaxation and low back flexibility.

64. MONKEY SLUMP

Stand with feet well apart, knees bent, hands on knees, head erect. Take a deep breath. Exhale slowly, letting the hands and upper body drop downward between the legs until the backs of the hands touch the floor. Attempt total relaxation of the upper body. Hang in the slumped position for a few seconds and return *slowly* to starting position while inhaling.

Adj – B/P: Do from a seated position.

Reps: 6

Purpose: Relaxation.

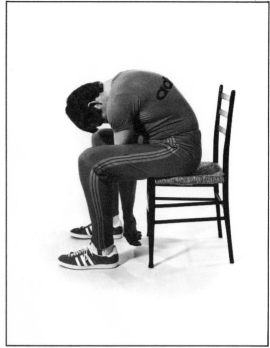

63. Seated Bent Over Sag

65. CATERPILLAR CRAWL

Sit with feet flat on floor, heels directly below knees. Stretch toes as far forward as possible and curl them slightly to drag foot forward in a caterpillar action. Pull with the pads of the toes; do not "claw" them underneath the foot. Crawl out as far as you can, then crawl back by pushing the foot back with the pads of the toes. You can do one foot at a time or both feet together.

Reps: 3x6 to 3x10   **Rest:** 10

Purpose: Strengthens muscles of the longitudinal arch.

66. ARCH LIFT AND HOLD

Sit with feet flat on floor. Lift arch of foot as high as you can. Hold for 5 seconds, relax and repeat. Do not curl toes under – keep pads on the floor.

Reps: 2x6   **Rest:** 10

Purpose: Strengthens muscles of the longitudinal arch.

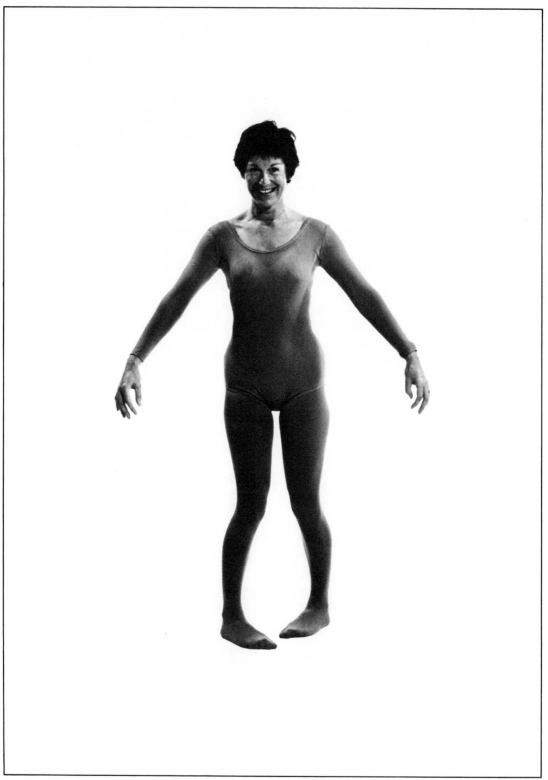

68. *Pigeon-toed Step Over*

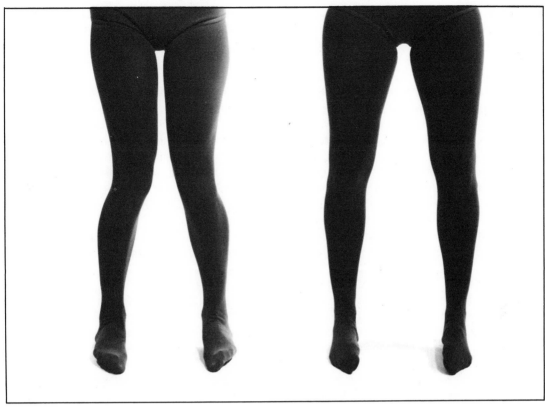

70. Foot Roll

67. MARBLE PICK UP

From a standing or sitting position, pick up a marble or bead with your toes. Hold for 3 to 5 seconds, drop it and repeat with other foot.

Reps: 2x6 to 2x10   **Rest:** 10

Purpose: Strengthens muscles of the metatarsal arch.

68. PIGEON-TOED STEP OVER

Stand with feet as pigeon-toed as possible. Walk with short steps, lifting one foot directly over the other, placing big toe on floor first. Do not walk on the outsides of the feet.

Reps: 3x10 to 3x20   **Rest:** 15

Purpose: Strengthens muscles and arches of the foot.

69. ROCK AND LIFT

Stand with feet hip-width apart. Rock back on your heels as far as you can without losing balance. Hold for 5 seconds, then rock forward onto tiptoes and hold for 5 seconds.

Reps: 8 to 12

Purpose: Strengthens muscles of foot and lower leg and improves balance.

70. FOOT ROLL

Stand with feet comfortably apart. Slowly shift weight to insides of feet, and then back to the outside. Move slowly and deliberately using the knees only slightly.

Reps: 2x10 to 2x20   **Rest:** 15

Purpose: Strengthens arches of the feet.

OTHER ACTIVITIES TO ENJOY

The perfect answer to the problem of keeping fit is to be so active physically that special exercises become unnecessary. This is particularly true for those individuals who hate calisthenics. Some people cannot abide the programmed route to fitness; they would rather remain sedentary. Almost all of us sooner or later become bored with a daily round of sit ups and knee bends, and it becomes a test of willpower to keep going.

This is why sports and active pastimes such as hiking or dancing should be a part of everyone's life style. They usually are not the complete answer, but they certainly increase the joy of movement and provide incentives to be creatively active throughout the year.

The sports approach usually falls down for the following reasons: 1. The activity has to be done regularly throughout the year. 2. It has to be intense enough to give the cardiovascular system a thorough workout. 3. It has to be varied enough to provide a certain amount of strength and flexibility training for the body. Too many activities are seasonal and not as intense and varied as they should be to promote total fitness.

Jogging and cycling, for example, are excellent for leg strength and heart-lung-circulatory fitness but fail to provide flexibility and upper body strength. Golf promotes flexibility, muscle sense, coordination and balance, but does little for the heart and lungs unless you happen to be eccentric enough to run between shots. Gymnastics is possibly the greatest all-round physical developer, but how many people have the skills to maintain a program of acrobatics throughout their lives?

Furthermore, most individuals are weekend athletes, confining their activities to Saturday and Sunday. Such infrequent exercise can be stressful, particularly if the sport is a violent one. Ideally, the body should have regular, moderate exercise, not intermittent high-frequency jolts.

Seasons create another handicap. There's not much point in playing tennis five times a week all summer and then letting the whole program fall apart in winter.

If your sports activity provides enough motivation for midweek practice and training, however, its value will be boosted immeasurably. Competitive sport should play a larger role in our lives, since rivalry is a stimulus for regular training. Industrialized societies often fail their citizens; a few elite athletes play for the benefit of huge audiences who watch on television but do not participate.

There is a tendency to blame ''elitism'' for this situation, but the reasons would appear to go deeper. Many school programs are not set up to develop skills in sports (badminton, tennis, orienteering, cross-country skiing) which can easily be continued once school days are over; nor is there machinery in place to enable the average high school hockey, football or baseball player to continue competition at an appropriate level of skill and intensity.

If you're active in sports and want to make sure you are getting maximum fitness benefits, it's a simple matter to determine your needs by taking the tests suggested earlier. If your sport or activity is not suitable to train certain weak spots which the tests may reveal, you should supplement it by developing a simple exercise program to be done two or three times a week. If your sport is seasonal, consider adopting a second sport or shifting your off-season emphasis to an exercise program. Even trained athletes find it difficult to get back in shape if they let themselves go between seasons, more so as they get older. Creating fitness is always harder than maintaining it.

Following is a brief rundown on a few of the common activities you should consider making a part of your life style. Remember not to let your enthusiasm run away with you at the start. Stay well within your capabilities, and build gradually. Watch for signs of over-stress: puffy or inflamed joints, chronic soreness, or sharp, stabbing pains in the muscles and tendons. These are all indications that you are trying to do too much, too soon.

WALKING

In this, the era of the jogger, many people consider walking a loafer's game. Not so. While a leisurely amble through the countryside may provide little more than fresh air, *real* walking is an excellent fitness activity.

As a matter of fact, it can do almost as much for your fitness as jogging, with less strain on joints and muscles. This is a particularly important point to remember for those who are in the middle-age bracket. The overweight, underexercised person of 40-or-over who suddenly tries to change a sedentary life style by becoming a jogger frequently winds up with little more than sore calves, swollen ankles, inflamed tendons and a depressed state of mind.

Swedish physiologists Per-Olof Astrand and Bengt Saltin measured the maximal oxygen uptake of Swedish competitive walking teams in 1967 and found that walkers averaged just over 70 millilitres per minute per kilogram of bodyweight. While long-distance runners were slightly higher, such athletes as rowers (63 ml/kg x min), swimmers and 400-metre runners (67 ml/kg x min) and wrestlers (57 ml/kg x min) were somewhat lower.

Not bad for the humble walker, but not so surprising when you consider that vigorous walking with a good arm action and a strong thrust off the toes involves some 150 pairs of muscles. The key word is "vigorous".

A competitive walker can sustain a pace of 8 miles an hour for 10 miles, which is faster than most of us can jog. For the average person 4 to 5 miles an hour would be a more reasonable pace. At 5 mph, you're burning up more than 550 calories per hour, and by using a variety of walking methods and techniques you can increase the load and create a greater general conditioning response.

Unfortunately, though, walking is a lost art. A well-organized person can get through the day without taking more than 15 or 20 long strides if he is careful to make maximum use of cars, elevators, and escalators.

If you can change that pattern — avoid cars

HOW WALKING BURNS UP CALORIES

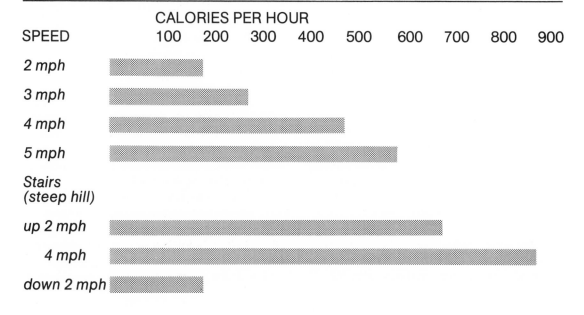

CALORIES PER HOUR

SPEED	100	200	300	400	500	600	700	800	900
2 mph									
3 mph									
4 mph									
5 mph									
Stairs (steep hill)									
up 2 mph									
4 mph									
down 2 mph									

where possible and walk up stairs instead of riding – you'll have taken a step in the right direction. If you use your walking as a fitness activity to get maximum benefits from it, you'll be well on the road to increased physical efficiency without increased stress.

One of the great advantages of walking as a fitness procedure is enjoyment. (This applies equally to cycling, swimming, cross-country skiing and similar activities.) If time is a problem, you may have to confine yourself to your own neighborhood and walk around the block a few times. The real pleasure comes from getting out in the country, even if only on weekends.

When that walk around the block can be converted into a hike along country roads and through the fields, taking the hills in stride without fatigue, you'll remember what it was like to be young.

1. Continuous Walking Set yourself an objective, a specific distance or a specific time. Start by covering it at an easy pace to establish your norm. Boost your pace every few days. Keep track of progress by measuring distance or time. This will give you a mark to shoot at during your fitness campaign.

2. Interval Walking Walk easily for 30 seconds, briskly for 30 seconds, and repeat until reasonably tired. Progress by increasing the number of easy-brisk intervals and/or length of brisk intervals. Every few workouts, test yourself against norm established in continuous walking.

3. Tempo Walking Warm up by walking easily for 5 minutes. Then walk at top speed for a minute. Every few workouts, add 5 seconds of top-speed walking. Cool off by walking easily for 5 minutes.

4. Long Stride Walk Insert into the 3 methods of walking described above a period or periods during which you walk with the longest possible stride. This will help condition the hips and buttocks.
Adj. – B: Shorten length of stride and lean well forward.

5. Hill Walking Warm up with 5 minutes of easy walking on the flat. Walk briskly up a small hill, and come back down slowly. Repeat until moderately tired. Cool off with an easy 5-minute walk on the flat. The out-of-condition individual should use discretion in selecting the steepness of hill. If a hill is not available, use stairs.

6. Military Walking Walk briskly with a highly emphasized arm action and a short, snappy stride. Use continuous, interval and tempo methods.

7. Stationary Walking Walk on the spot, lifting the knees as high as possible. Start at an easy pace and gradually increase speed. Use continuous, interval, and tempo methods.

8. Variety Walking Use a variety of the above walking methods, changing over from day to day. This will give you the advantages of all the systems outlined here and will provide some variety for your program.

Remember to keep track of progress by measuring yourself against the norm you've established in continuous walking.

JOGGING

In the past few years, thanks to Aerobics and some other excellent programs, jogging has become possibly the single most-used fitness activity in North America. It is inexpensive, simple, and provides the most dividends for the least effort, particularly for heart-circulatory fitness which is probably the most important element of our physical machine.

However, jogging is not to everyone's taste. It's a sad fact that the poorer your heart-wind fitness, the less you're likely to enjoy jogging. Further, some people are simply not equipped psychologically to jog. They do it, but they don't like it. It bores them. Eventually, unless they have formidable willpower, they drift back to the TV set and a sedentary life style.

Moreover, jogging can cause foot and leg problems for the over-40-year-old who hasn't exercised in years. He or she starts off with a burst of enthusiasm, dismisses those early aches and pains as "shin splints", and ends up with chronic muscle strain, swollen ankles, or foot problems.

It doesn't have to be that way; there's a right and a wrong way to jog.

Some joggers land on the ball of the foot, then allow the heel to touch the ground before pushing off into the next stride. This is fine for sprinters and quarter-milers, but most middle and long-distance runners use a heel-toe action because it's more economical and places less strain on the foot and achilles tendon.

Since jogging is a form of distance running, it makes sense to use a heel-toe action. In cases of foot and leg soreness the ball-heel foot action is often the culprit. It throws a strain on the arches of the foot and the muscles in the calf, which are required to absorb the shock as the full weight of the body lands on the foot. When the jogger changes to a heel landing, the condition usually clears up.

The secret is to develop a "soft" knee. The shock of landing must be absorbed by the flexed knee (never land on a straight leg). Some runners have the knack instinctively; others tend to land heavily and must concentrate on getting the "feel" of that soft landing in which the ankles are flexible and the knees bend slightly as they take up the weight of the body.

The jogger should also make sure his shoes have a well-padded heel. If you are a naturally "heavy" runner, you'd be wise to get special inserts for your heels, or cut foam rubber to fit in your running shoes. Where possible, run on a grassy surface rather than a road or a track.

Finally, the way you start your jogging program can have lasting effects.

Those of us who are ex-athletes remember how we used to run — like antelopes, or so it seems now. When we start jogging it all comes back. We're as good as we ever were, for the first few strides, at least.

But, common sense should tell us that the tendons and muscles aren't as flexible and strong as they used to be. They'll respond for a while, but if you try to do too much too soon you'll probably acquire all kinds of foot and leg complaints. Too many jogging programs end in the first week for that reason.

It is better to do far less than you think you can for the first month or two. Concentrate on developing a soft, relaxed running technique; don't be too anxious to start building toward maximum effort. That will come, but your legs will be much better for the easy start.

A few minor aches and pains are nothing to worry about, particularly along the shins. They should go away fairly soon. Watch carefully for any sharp pains, and if your aches seem to be building up day by day, don't try to simply run through them. Take a few days off, and reduce your exercise intensity when you start again. It's probably a warning from your tendons and muscles that they're being overstressed and that the adaptive response of the body is unequal to the demands you are making of it.

There are several ways you can jog. You may want a nice easy run one day, and perhaps some interval work the next; or a combination of the two. You may want to do some station training — jogging a bit, doing an exercise, running or jogging some more, doing another exercise, and so on. There are even special courses for this, known as Vita Parcours.

Jogging is great for the heart, wind, and circulation as well as for strength and muscle endurance of the legs, lower back, and abdomen. It's also excellent relaxation activity if done properly. Good track and field runners have a loose, fluid movement which you should be trying to develop.

The arms and shoulders should swing freely and easily – you can feel the shoulder muscles loosen as you run. At the same time an easy, upright carriage of the head and chest is important to allow the respiratory muscles full play and to develop the so-called holding muscles of the upper body. But no muscle that isn't actually working should be in tension when you are running, and you should be consciously attempting to keep all parts of your body – hands, arms, shoulders, jaw, upper and lower legs, ankles – as relaxed as you can.

At the beginning of your program, jog for 50 yards, walk for 50 yards, run 50 more and so on until you feel pleasurably tired. Then walk until fully recovered. No need to push too hard. That can come later.

After a week or two build up the length of the jog, without increasing the walk, until the jog-walk ratio is about two to one. Now you can start to add extra intervals, and perhaps boost your jogging speed.

Improvise your own program, using fatigue and inclination as the measure of how much you do. Be guided by your body's reactions, including the response of the leg and foot muscles as you increase the stress. Eventually, you'll be in shape to get in shape. Now you can begin to push yourself with some confidence that all the components are going to hold together despite a fairly strong workload.

Once your easy jogging program has tuned up your body and legs to the point where you can handle a mile at a steady pace with your heart beat in the training rate range discussed on page 61, you'll be ready to follow your own inclinations. Try to maintain this workload for at least 15 minutes each day, although you don't have to run at a steady pace for that long. Three intervals of five minutes of running, with a couple of minutes of walking in between, will have almost the same effect.

Having measurable standards is a good idea in jogging, as well as in the rest of your fitness activities. Measure out a course, even if you only pace it out. When you're in shape to handle it, time yourself over that course. Every month or so, have a time trial to see how you're progressing. Don't try to set new world records; run at the fastest pace you are able to handle without excessive stress.

Always remember to cool down after a hard workout or time trial with 10 to 15 minutes of easy, relaxed jogging and walking. It helps the heart and circulation to return to normal faster and with less strain, and it also enables the blood stream to disperse lactic acid and other fatigue products which cause muscle soreness.

Hill running is excellent cardiovascular and leg strength work. If you can find a long hill, so much the better. On a smaller hill, do interval training once a week – run up, walk down, and repeat as able.

When you can't get outdoors, you can jog on the spot. Here, a ball of the foot landing must be used. Remember to keep the knees and ankles loose. Include some high-knee running and ''sprinting'' if you want to boost your work load.

You can increase the relaxation-inducing quality of your jogging by doing a tight-loose drill which helps to teach your muscles the ''feeling'' of relaxation. Tighten the muscles of your arms and shoulders for a few seconds as you jog along, then let them become lax; feel the relaxation seep into them as you move. Repeat several times at intervals during your run. The same technique can be used with the legs, stomach, and other parts of the body.

The body may be unable to cope with residual tension because it doesn't recognize that it's there. So say to yourself as you do this tight-loose drill: ''This is tension, this is what it feels like'', and then, ''My shoulder muscles are relaxed; this is what it feels like.'' Try to key your mind and body to a conscious recognition of the difference between relaxation and tension. This simple biofeedback technique will help you reach that wonderful stage where the muscles start to relax automatically in response to tension and tension-producing situations.

A final point to remember. Jogging or any other strenuous activity done only once a week can be a source of stress, especially for older persons. If you're going to jog, three times a week is a minimum. You can skip a week here or there if it's necessary or occasionally do only one workout during the week. However, the weekend jogger, skier, or swimmer can't expect much return in improved fitness.

SWIMMING

Like walking, swimming can vary greatly in the fitness benefits it provides. If you merely float about for a while, you probably won't get much more out of it than cleanliness. If you're interested in getting fit, it *can* do a lot for your heart-circulatory-respiratory system, your overall muscular strength, flexibility and posture, and mental relaxation.

There are three basic methods you can use to develop fitness:

1. Tempo swimming – a series of fast bursts with full recovery rest periods between each one.

2. Interval swimming – longer bursts at a moderately fast pace with intervals of easy, relaxed swimming in between.

3. Continuous swimming for long distances.

You may find interval swimming the most enjoyable method, although tempo swimming may have an edge for development of strength and endurance. Try all three systems, and mix up your strokes to make sure that all the muscle groups get a workout.

Done methodically, swimming will develop even more areas of the body than jogging.

However it does have some drawbacks. Unfortunately not everybody has a lake or a pool within easy reach, and some people dislike the chlorinated water and lack of variety in doing lengths in a pool. Swimming is less beneficial for the joints than weight-bearing activities such as walking or jogging.

GOLF

Golf tends to be fairly mild exercise, since the walking involved is generally not fast enough to benefit heart-wind efficiency. A hilly course can give you a good workout, however. Always carry your own bag and never use a motorized cart.

Since most courses are between 6,600 and 6,900 yards in length, a normal rate of play will use up between 250 and 300 calories per hour. Useful enough, as long as you don't regain that and more at the 19th hole.

Golf is a good activity for upper body and hip flexibility, coordination, balance, and muscle sense (sometimes called kinesthetic sense). It is a useful tension release, provided that you are not one of those highly competitive individuals who play too intensely and are easily frustrated.

DANCING

Dancing regularly and vigorously can provide a great workout; but few of us go dancing three times a week, which is the minimum requirement for progressive fitness.

However, doing exercises rhythmically to music takes away much of the drudgery so frequently associated with fitness exercises, and is relaxing as well.

Music with a strong beat – jazz, pop, rock – stimulates the desire to move; there is an accompanying physiological and psychological upsurge. Experiment to find tempos that fit your particular program.

CYCLING

Like walking, jogging, swimming, and similar activities, cycling is excellent for heart-wind fitness and leg strength and endurance if it is tackled as a training activity. Use interval and tempo training systems, as well as continuous cycling. Try to include some hills in your workout.

Flexibility exercises, particularly for the back thighs, should be a part of your fitness program if you choose cycling as your activity.

PADDLING, ROWING

Done agressively, paddling and rowing provide excellent conditioning for the heart and upper body, and rowing also benefits the leg muscles. Use interval and tempo training as well as continuous work for maximum results.

SKIING (DOWNHILL)

Downhill skiing is overrated as a fitness activity, particularly if it is done only on weekends. The risks probably outweigh the benefits. It will develop leg, hip, and abdominal strength and can be a good fitness activity if you participate in pre-season training, and ski at least three times per week.

SKIING (CROSS-COUNTRY)

One of the best fitness activities of all, particularly if tackled vigorously, is cross-country skiing. An excellent heart-wind-circulatory exercise, it develops strength and endurance in the arms and shoulders as well as the legs, improves balance, and helps to release tension. Oxygen uptake of top competitive cross-country skiers is the highest measured in any sport.

For best results use both interval and continuous approaches – as in walking and jogging – and plenty of uphill work as well.

Cross-country skiing can be stressful if you ski only on weekends. A midweek workout or two is required to keep in condition.

BOWLING, CURLING

These mild forms of exercise contribute little to fitness. However, they can offer good tension-relieving recreation. The sweepers in curling will benefit from the upper body workout, although it is usually not continuous enough to provide top level conditioning.

BADMINTON, TENNIS, SQUASH, HANDBALL

All are good heart-wind conditioners, since they involve a lot of leg work. They are also useful for developing shoulder and upper body flexibility, and tennis in particular strengthens the racket arm and shoulder.

The player should learn to regulate his activity to match his level of fitness. Build slowly if you are out of condition. If you are an older person, be cautious in strenuous play – the foot, ankle and leg muscles, tendons and ligaments will not take the pounding they were able to withstand when you were young. Treat aches and pains with respect and get a medical check if you notice a tendency to chronic soreness, sharp knifelike pains, or swollen ankles.

SKIPPING ROPE

Skipping rope is great for cardiovascular fitness and leg strength. It does not have much value for the upper body, however, unless you swing the rope with a full overhead arm extension from the shoulders.

Start slowly, and precede your skipping with some flexibility exercises. You can skip at a steady speed, or you can use the interval system: short bursts of high-speed skipping with rest periods in between. Check your pulse for training effect, as advised in Chapter 3. If you skip at a good rate, there's strong evidence that you can accomplish as much in 15 minutes as you can with 30 minutes of jogging.

In addition to normal skipping technique, insert variety and increase the conditioning element for the legs by skipping on one leg only, first the left, then the right. Do some jumping as well, trying to get as high as you can in the air with each leap. See how many times you can get the rope around before you land.

GARDENING

This mild form of exercise involves some muscular activity, particularly for the upper body, but very little heart-wind conditioning. Digging can provide a good overall workout, but may be dangerous for persons with high blood pressure and heart problems. The major benefits of gardening are in relieving tension.

Beware of heavy lifting if you're not in good condition, and always start easily when you first get outdoors in the spring. Many a back has been sprung by the early burst of enthusiasm to which the body is unequal after a winter of inactivity.

RIDING

A mild form of exercise which provides some internal massage. Stimulating and refreshing when done as recreation, but not much use in developing heart-wind fitness. Better you should walk.

VOLLEYBALL

This sport can provide a pretty good workout, if you're fit enough to enter into all the leaping, diving, and tumbling. If not, regard it as fun and relaxing, but not much of a conditioner.

DIFFICULTIES YOU MAY ENCOUNTER

When you start to exercise, your body complains. It aches, it gets stiff, muscles sometimes cramp up and joints crackle. Although these symptoms are usually minor

and pass with time and perseverance, sometimes they are significant and should be checked by a doctor. The problem lies in knowing which is which — you don't want to rush to your physician every time a muscle goes into spasm, but you'd like to know what's happening.

This section may help alleviate some of your anxieties about muscle soreness, cramps, stitches, shin splints, creaky joints, blackouts, and exercise during hot weather or pregnancy.

Many physical symptoms of stress are not merely the result of lack of fitness. Even a well-conditioned individual may experience a reaction to any sudden change in activity. You may, for example, be able to run a mile in six minutes and still wind up with sore muscles after a hard session of squash or downhill skiing.

Muscle Soreness

Muscular aches are a part of physical activity and are virtually impossible to avoid. They are a badge you can wear with a certain amount of pride before your sedentary friends. Privately, however, you suffer. What can you do about it?

There are three types of muscle soreness. One is caused by a sudden increase in activity levels, and can be relieved by taking a short rest. The second strikes anywhere from 12 to 48 hours after the activity ends. The third is caused by injury: a strain or a tear.

The second type of muscle soreness is the most common. It can mean two things: 1. You're out of shape and you'll just have to grin and bear it. Continuing mild exercise will help it to disappear in time, but if you've done too much too soon your muscles may feel sore and tired for several weeks. 2. You're increasing the intensity of your program too quickly. If you are getting too much muscle soreness you should ease off on the frequency/duration/intensity of your exercises.

If you suffer a muscle injury, treatment will depend on severity. For very mild strains with no apparent internal bleeding – the "bruised" appearance caused by a muscle strain—the best treatment usually is to keep using the muscle, but very gently. Build up intensity over a period of several days. This will help the circulation aid the body's natural restoration processes.

However, if the injury is fairly severe and is accompanied by a spreading bruised patch at the point of strain, apply cold compresses (ice wrapped in towels) as soon as you can. This will help to reduce internal bleeding. The next day, bathe it several times for 20 or 30 minutes in hot compresses to increase circulation. For such injuries, most doctors skilled in sports medicine also advocate very gentle exercise starting the day following the injury, building gradually as the muscle regains strength. You will be very stiff at first, but the muscle should gradually loosen up as you use it.

If your return to mild exercise seems to restart the internal bleeding, or causes sudden sharp pains, postpone activity for a day or two.

Never massage such an injury in its early stages, as this may aggravate the internal bleeding. If the strain is so severe you lose the use of the limb, have it checked by a doctor.

Remember, too, that it's important to warm up properly before starting the strenuous part of your program. Equally vital is the cool off period. If you stop suddenly, the fatigue products may not be properly dispersed. Residual lactic acid can irritate the nervous system. Decelerate. Keep moving for 15 to 20 minutes. A warm bath or shower will help too.

Specificity of exercise plays a part in muscle soreness. You may be in great shape to jog 5 miles, but try playing tennis and because of the new, unaccustomed movements the muscles of your upper body and arms will start to ache. Begin slowly whenever you switch to new and different physical exertions.

Static stretching will ease some forms of muscle soreness. Stretch the muscle or muscles which are sore as slowly as possible, and without too much force. Hold the maximum stretch for about 2 minutes (the static position), relax for a few seconds, and repeat 6 or 7 times.

Chronic muscle soreness may signal a medical condition, and should be examined by a doctor.

Cramps

Like muscle soreness, cramps can be caused by sudden increases in activity levels, and/or residual lactic acid deposits. Treatment is similar in both cases: continued activity, concentration on warm up and cool off, and static stretching of the cramped muscle. Cramps can also be caused by a blow on a muscle.

Some people seldom get cramps. Others suffer from them a great deal. The reasons for these individual differences are still somewhat vague, although they have been traced to diet (shortages of calcium, potassium and magnesium) and body type. Tense individuals may be more prone to cramps than those who are relaxed.

Lack of salt and fluids can be responsible for cramps. If you perspire a lot, drink plenty of water and use salt generously with your food. Taking salt tablets is not a good idea because the sudden introduction of excessive salt into the system can also cause problems.

When a cramp strikes, do not use a sudden, bouncing type of stretching exercise to relieve it. This can invoke the so-called myotatic reflex in which the muscle responds by going into further spasm. Stretch *slowly*, and hold for two minutes or until you can relax without the muscle's cramping up again. Gentle massage (no vigorous pounding) may also help.

Some authorities feel older people should finish every workout with a session of static stretching in order to guard against cramps and muscle soreness.

Shin Splints

Shin splits are a particularly annoying form of muscle soreness which almost everyone has experienced at one time or another. Opinion is widely divided as to the exact reason, but we all know the result: stiff, sore areas along the inside or the outside of the shinbones above the ankles.

Sometimes shin splints react to rest, sometimes they don't. Sometimes they signal deeper problems, such as a stress fracture. Occasionally they can become an inflamed, chronic condition which makes even walking a painful experience.

Let's look at some of the more common causes:

1. Training, jogging or even walking too vigorously and for too long, relative to the fitness of the muscles. This usually occurs at the start of a training campaign, but it can happen at any time.

2. Jolting shocks to the muscle in jumping or landing too hard on unyielding surfaces when jogging, especially when the legs are not in good condition. Can be caused by poor running technique, stiff ankle or knee action, overstriding, landing on the inside of foot instead of the outside, or wearing shoes with insufficient cushioning in the heel.

3. Lack of flexibility in the calf muscles and achilles tendons.

4. Running on the ball of the foot for long periods. Joggers beware—use a heel-toe action.

5. Arch troubles. Shin splints may signify that an arch is dropping.

6. Shoes too loose, or too tight, causing a change in foot-strike and throwing an unaccustomed strain on the shock-absorbing muscles.

7. Weakness of the lower leg muscles.

8. Inadequate warm up.

9. One leg slightly shorter than the other. Ask someone to check if your ankle bones are exactly opposite each other as you lie on your back. If legs are uneven in length, a small pad or lift in one heel of your running shoes may help ease the problem.

Preventive measures include:

1. Strengthen and stretch the muscles of the lower leg with early season exercises. These might be: walking on your heels; lifting weighted objects with your toes; stretching the calves by leaning against a wall on your hands and slowly pressing the heels to the ground as far back behind you as you can; rocking back and forth from your toes to your heels; lifting the toes of one foot while pressing down on them with the other foot (sit in a chair to do this one).

2. Concentrate on using a "soft" landing when jogging. Ankles and knees should be loose to take up the shock. Jog on grass rather than on hard surfaces. Use a good heel cushion in your shoes.

3. Start gradually. A vigorous beginning to a jogging or hiking program will frequently cause shin splints.

4. Avoid long walks in new shoes, especially those with thick, inflexible soles.

5. Start treatment early.

TREATMENT

1. Following your workout, soak your lower legs in hot water for 15 to 20 minutes. Use a hot pack (a thin layer of vaseline, followed by an analgesic balm covered with a loose bandage) overnight while you sleep.

2. Follow the preventive measures suggested above. Ease off on exercise intensity for a few days.

3. Rest, if these measures do not work. If shin splints do not respond, check with your physician for possible complications.

4. Make sure you warm up and cool off properly.

5. Avoid vigorous massage; it will usually intensify the problem. Light surface massage may help, however.

Creaky Joints

People often worry about the noises emanating from their joints during exercise: creaks, cracks, and pops, sometimes loud enough to be heard several feet away. Relax. It's a common occurrence.

If there is no pain or discomfort associated with the popping, carry on exercising. The problem could be due to a lack of lubricating fluid in the joint, or it could be caused by the movement of tendons or ligaments over a bony protuberance as the joint bends.

Make sure you warm up properly; the heat created during warm ups helps to start arms and legs moving smoothly.

If there is some discomfort accompanying the popping noises, a medical problem might exist: a bone spur building up around an old injury, a problem with the cartilage, or a separation. Check with your doctor. The stiff upper lip and "press on regardless" attitude could result in damage.

Exercise and Hot Weather

Sweating is the mechanism the body uses to help regulate internal temperature during physical activity, particularly when the weather is hot. Vigorous activity during especially hot days carries with it certain hazards, and it's best to be familiar with them in order to avoid excessive fatigue, loss of skill, and possibly heat exhaustion or heat stroke.

First, you become dehydrated. This is obvious. An athlete may sweat off 10 pounds or more during a single afternoon. This loss can and should be replaced as soon as possible. Gone are the days when athletes were ordered not to drink during practices and games; many top coaches now make it compulsory to take small amounts at intervals during strenuous workouts.

Along with liquids, we lose a considerable amount of salt and other elements such as potassium and magnesium. Rather than relying on the old-fashioned salt pill (too much salt ingested suddenly can be bad), sprinkle extra salt on your food, or drink salted vegetable juice, consomme or some other beverage.

If you are going to be involved in strenuous activity during hot, humid weather, make up a mixture containing half a teaspoon of salt to a quart of liquid (water, tomato juice). Drink about 10 ounces half an hour before activity starts, and every 20 to 30 minutes during activity as well. Afterwards, replenish your body with plenty of fluids, especially fruit and vegetable juices, consomme or tea.

Cool drinks are better than cold ones. While you may think you get more relief from a cold drink, the body actually produces *more* heat to compensate, and in the long run you will feel hotter than ever.

Stitches

While they may not concur as to the cause, most doctors do agree on the *definition* of the side stitch: a muscle spasm causing pain on one side of the abdomen or lower chest during exercise. Dr. D. Sinclair of the University of Auckland Medical School in New Zealand found that for a stitch to occur, there usually had to be recurrent vertical jolts to the body, such as those sustained in cycling or motorcycling over rough terrain, playing basketball, tennis or football, and running or jogging. Swimmers or rowers seldom had stitches.[1]

Dr. Sinclair theorized from his findings that the side stitch was the result of mechanical stress which stretched the peritoneal ligaments. These are attached to the diaphragm and support the liver, spleen, or stomach. Hence the higher incidence of stitches with a full stomach or weak stomach muscles.

If recurring stitches are a problem for you, make sure you wait an hour or two after meals before exercising heavily, and do stomach-strengthening exercises.

If you do get a stitch, Dr. Sinclair suggests that you breathe in deeply and bend forward, pressing your hand against the affected area. Breathe in and out normally while maintaining pressure for a few seconds. This should help to relax the peritoneal ligaments and relieve the pain.

Blackouts

If you've been sitting or lying down for some time or exercising vigorously in a prone position, you may find on standing up suddenly that the world goes blank. You think you're going to faint. What's happening?

Most people have experienced blackouts. (They may well occur at the start of an intensive fitness program.) The cause usually is simple: a temporary shortage of blood to the brain.

During vigorous exercise blood is "borrowed" by the working muscles. At rest, 15 per cent of the body's total blood supply is being distributed to the brain, with another 15 to 20 per cent going to the muscles. During exercise the blood circulates faster and the muscles' share may jump to 85 per cent, while the flow to the brain falls to 2 or 3 per cent.

If you stop exercising suddenly, some of the blood will tend to remain in the dilated blood vessels within the muscles of the arms and legs. Blood pressure may drop and the brain will be temporarily "starved".

This pooling of the blood may also occur when you lie or sit in one position for a period of time. The flow of blood to the heart for recirculation to the lungs is reduced; the heart reacts by cutting back on its output and arterial blood pressure is lowered. The fall in pressure does not become significant until you stand up. Then there is an immediate increase in heart rate, a further slight decrease in blood pressure as the heart starts pumping up blood from the legs to the lungs, and a shortage of oxygen-supplying red cells in the brain. You feel faint or dizzy.

A soldier standing at attention for a long time, particularly in hot weather or after a long march, often gets the same pooling effect. A person playing tennis or badminton may have an attack if he or she stops suddenly and stands still.

If you do feel faint, lie down with the legs raised. This should restore proper circulation.

This blackout phenomenon is one more reason for warming up and cooling off properly before and after hard activity. Both help the body adapt to the various changes in blood flow which must take place.

Exercise and Pregnancy

Should pregnant women continue vigorous exercise? Evidence is that they should, and that if there are no obstetrical complications, it will be extremely beneficial.

A study of Hungarian athletes indicated that they had shorter periods of labor, quicker delivery, and that there were 50 per cent fewer Caesarean deliveries than in a comparable group of sedentary mothers.

Sports & Fitness Instructor quoted Dr. Lindsay A. Belch, chief of gynecology and obstetrics at North York General Hospital: "With a normal pregnancy there is no reason why a patient cannot continue to do all the activities she is used to doing and doing well, providing these activities are not carried out to the point of excessive fatigue or muscle strain. There is no reason a good tennis player should not continue to play tennis during pregnancy, although it's not a good idea for a woman to take up competitive tennis at this time if she's never played before. Swimming is good exercise which can be continued up to close term."[2]

How much should she do? It depends on the individual. According to Dr. Belch there will be no harm in carrying on normal exercise until the sixth or seventh month. Walking and swimming can continue much further.

However, he warns: "You shouldn't try to

make athletes out of all women just because they are pregnant. If you take someone who weighs 240 lbs. — who shouldn't be pregnant anyway — she's better off with a program of walking or swimming than trying to do pushups.''

As always, you should be guided by your family physician. But here's a final point to remember from Dr. Belch.

''It should be strongly stressed that physical preparation for childbirth should start *before* a woman gets pregnant. The woman who puts on 40 or 50 lbs. of weight during pregnancy and allows her muscles to get out of tone and thinks she'll lose the weight after the pregnancy, because she feels she can't do it during pregnancy, is wrong. Usually, she does not.

''I think women who are physically fit tolerate their labor better, have a smoother convalescence and a more rapid return to normal afterwards.''

6

Special Problems

HOW TO REPAIR PHYSICAL FAULTS

Strength, endurance, or a feeling of youth and vigor are all important reasons why you may have decided to get fit. But there's another, equally valid source of motivation: the desire to remedy a physical fault which is either causing pain or spoiling your appearance.

The appeal may be to simple vanity, but the implications often go deeper than that. Many developing physical imperfections are symptoms of more serious trouble on the horizon. Today's sagging stomach muscles which are embarassing you on the beach may be tomorrow's back pain or digestive difficulty.

Anyone, man or woman, with particular physical problems, especially spinal and abdominal abnormalities, should read this chapter and seriously consider the implications. While you may not give a damn whether your knees look knobby from behind, it should bother you if a sagging abdomen is ruining your silhouette, because the strain on your framework could have serious

implications for your health. Correcting physical defects is relevant to everyone's fitness.

Because of our sedentary life style, muscles sag, curves vanish, the body droops, and morale follows suit. But cheer up – if you're really bothered because you're not the person you used to be, there's still a lot you can do about it.

The shape you're in is probably due to three main causes. One is Mother Nature's Department of Dirty Tricks, the second is the aging process, and the third is your life style.

Your genetic endowment provides you with certain physical features, such as long legs or thin arms, or knobby knees. You can't do much about the length and bony protuberances of your limbs, but you can modify the way they're covered up. If you have thin arms, you can build muscle and form through proper exercise. If your joints are too prominent, you can help to disguise them by building up the muscle tissue around them. If your shoulder blades protude, you can try to improve your posture and increase the size of the back muscles so the wingbones don't show so much.

114

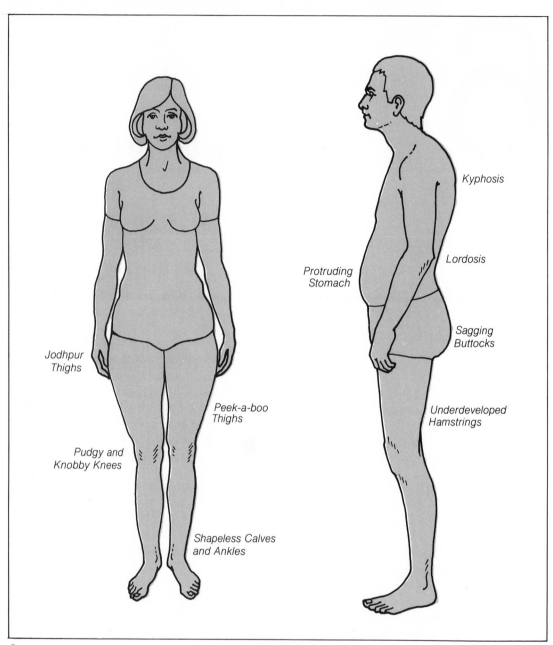

Special Problems

The battle against gravity begins as soon as you stop crawling and stand erect. As you get older, you start to lose the war. The muscles are no longer strong and flexible enough to maintain good posture, and the body's framework starts to bend. Older people are often startled to find they're an inch or two shorter than they were in their twenties — that's gravity at work.

You can accelerate the rate at which you lose your anti-gravity campaign by developing poor posture habits, by allowing your muscles to degenerate through sedentary living, and by carrying around excess fat which drags you down.

These three factors not only cause figure faults but affect your health as well. Since the organs are no longer held firmly in their proper places, they start to sag and lose tone along with the rest of the body. Some of them become cramped for space and their ability to function efficiently is impaired.

The parts of the body which appear to become disaster areas most often are the abdomen and buttocks, the upper body (head and shoulder slump), the knees and, in older persons, the underside of the upper arms. These problems seldom appear singly because the various segments are inextricably linked, and trouble in one area causes trouble somewhere else. Similarly , if you remedy a fault in one area, other areas will benefit as well.

People who have dieted to remove excess weight are often discouraged to find that their bodies don't immediately snap back into their old familiar shape, making dieting seem a waste of time and willpower. The fatty tissue has stretched the muscles and tendons slightly and when the dieting's done, the sag remains. This is particularly true of the gluteus maximus (buttock muscles), triceps (underside of the upper arms) and abdominals. Proper exercise can help to reduce this problem and perhaps eliminate it. Even if you're into your 50s and 60s, you can still firm up your muscles and restore much of their tone. A well-exercised, fit body radiates

its own particular chemistry. It has zest and energy; we hardly notice that it may be imperfect.

This chapter will examine some of the major fault lines in the body, and suggest the remedies that will help to put them right. To be 100 per cent effective, they usually should be associated with some form of weight control: a reduction in calorie intake if you're too fat, an increase in calories and other food elements if you're too slender. (See Chapter 7 on nutrition and weight control.)

Most of the exercises described here are resistance exercises involving muscular exertion against other muscles, or against weights. They are particularly effective in rapid strengthening of muscles and in establishing a fixed structural posture. In this sense, they are not "conditioning" exercises; if total fitness is your objective, make them part of an overall program such as the one outlined in Chapter 4.

For faster improvement, these exercises should be done more than once per day. If a sagging abdomen is your problem, for example, take a few minutes in the morning, a few minutes in the afternoon and again at night to do the particular exercise or exercises designed to do the job for that area.

To erase bulges and sags, do many repetitions of an exercise, using little resistance. To build up underdeveloped areas or disguise protruding bones, try fewer repetitions of each exercise but with greater resistance (more weight or greater muscular exertion).

Forget the old myth that building muscle bulk will produce bulges like an overblown shotputter's. The amount of work you would have to do to increase your proportions to that extent is staggering, even if you had the genetic endowment for it to happen — which most people do not.

During resistance exercise you may have a tendency to hold your breath. Try to breathe normally during the hold or resistance phase of each movement.

FEET

The human foot, according to Dr. Irwin Ross, a leading specialist, is one of the most ingenious and versatile devices ever designed. It serves as a cushion, support lever, hydraulic jack, and catapult. "Nature has successfully crammed an intricate, multi-purpose mechanism into a space smaller than that of a milk carton", says Dr. Ross. "The moving and supporting parts are 26 neatly intermeshed bones driven by millions of muscle fibers, nourished by a maze of blood vessels, coordinated by the electrical signals of thread-like nerves. The power supply consists of great, contracting muscles in the thighs and upper legs."[1]

Ingenious though it may be, many people suffer from foot problems. A lifetime of jumping up and down on 26 neatly intermeshed bones crammed into something nature would never have dreamed of designing causes a breakdown sooner or later.

Sensible, properly designed footwear is one answer. Fashion usually rules it out, however. Walking correctly is another: feet parallel instead of turned out, weight on the bones at the outside of the arch.

The third solution is exercises which will help relieve tired aching tendons and ligaments, start the circulation flowing again, and build up the strength of the arch-supporting muscles.

Exercises designed to do this are in Chapter 5, nos. 65 to 70.

LEGS

Your fitness program should include as much activity for the legs as you can give them without depriving other areas of their fair share. The biggest muscles and a tremendous number of blood vessels are located in the legs. When the legs are given vigorous work, there is an exceptionally

strong heart-circulatory response. It is difficult to get as effective heart-wind training with the smaller muscles of the arms alone, and therefore jogging, walking, cycling, tennis, cross-country skiing, and similar activities are central to a good fitness program.

In addition, the squat exercises found in Chapter 5, nos. 2 to 14, are excellent conditioners and strength developers, designed especially for the legs. If you are in poor shape, use only the first three (2, 3 and 4). Once you reach what you consider to be good condition, gradually include the rest. Start at a moderate tempo, and increase it as your strength and stamina improve. This will provide a conditioning effect. If strength is your primary concern, do them slowly (except for the squat jump) and use progressively heavier weights instead of increased tempo and repetitions.

For general toning and conditioning, the interval method is probably the best route to follow. Find out how many repetitions of the exercise you can do at one time without excessive fatigue. Then cut this in half and do 3 or 4 sets of the resulting figure with a 20-second rest in between. This will enable you to carry a heavier work load than simply doing one long set of your maximum repetitions.

Once every couple of weeks, see how many reps you can do, cut *this* number in half and use it as the basis for a new set of repetitions.

If your legs are exceptionally strong and well-conditioned, you may find you can handle a large number of repetitions. In this case, it's best to add resistance in the form of dumbbells or some other weight held in the hands, rather than spending a lot of time doing excessive numbers of reps.

The major faults of the legs are:

- Underdevelopment of the inner thighs (see-through or peek-a-boo thighs);
- Fatty or fleshy deposits on the outside of the upper thighs (saddlebags or jodhpur thighs);

- Flat, underdeveloped hamstrings (the group of muscles and their tendons located at the back of the thighs);
- Knobby or pudgy knees;
- Shapeless calves and ankles.

Let's look at these problems one by one.

Peek-a-boo Thighs

Stand in front of a full-length mirror with your feet close together and your knees touching. If there is a gap between the upper legs, you've got see-through thighs. When the inner thigh muscles (the adductors) which draw your legs together are properly developed, they fill out most of the inner thigh area so that there is no unsightly gap.

Fat may mask see-through thighs. If you've got that much of it, chances are your knees, hips, and waist have their share as well; so get it off and then check again. If you spot a gap, do the following exercises to encourage development of those vital adductor muscles:

 CUSHION SQUEEZE HALF SQUAT

Stand with feet about 12 inches apart. Holding a small, firm cushion between your knees and keeping heels flat on floor, sink into a half squat (Exercise 7) so that your upper legs are almost parallel to the floor. Return to starting position, exerting strong pressure on the cushion with your knees throughout the movement.

Reps: 3x6 to 3x20   **Rest:** 15 sec.

 SEATED KNEE PRESS

Sit on the edge of a chair with your feet flat on floor, 2 to 4 inches apart. Make fists with both hands and place them together (thumb to thumb) between your knees. Press your knees hard against your fists for 5 seconds, relax for 5 seconds, and repeat.

Reps: 10x5 sec. to 25x5 sec.
Rest: 5 seconds.

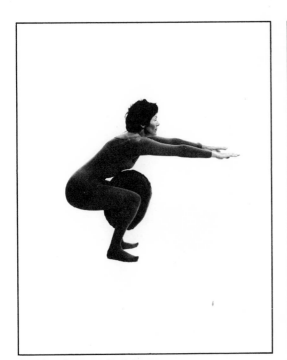

Cushion Squeeze Half Squat

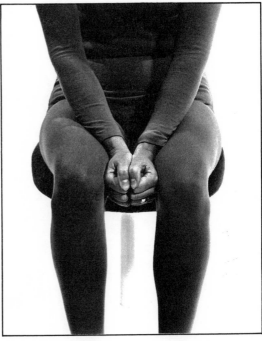

Seated Knee Press

Saddlebags

Jodhpur thighs frequently have nothing to do with obesity. Dieting may remove the fat but leave the saddlebags. If lack of consistent vigorous activity has allowed the buttock muscles to sag, the flesh on the sides of the thighs is pushed outward, causing those unsightly bulges. Sometimes, along with flabby stomach muscles, they are an unwelcome legacy from a pregnancy.

The exercises recommended in this chapter for the hips, waist, and buttocks will help to snap the gluteals back where they belong, and will tone up the area on the outside of the thighs. Fat won't readily collect in areas where circulation is good and muscle activity is high (but it won't disappear completely as long as you're overweight).

Hamstrings

This area is often neglected, yet the back of the thigh is an important part of a well-shaped leg. Sedentary living not only leads to a certain amount of hamstring atrophy but also causes the muscle to shorten and lose flexibility. When we stand, it no longer takes the shape nature intended it to. Fat also tends to congregate at the back of the thigh giving it a "puckered" look.

Useful exercises in Chapter 5 are nos. 43, 44, 45, and 53.

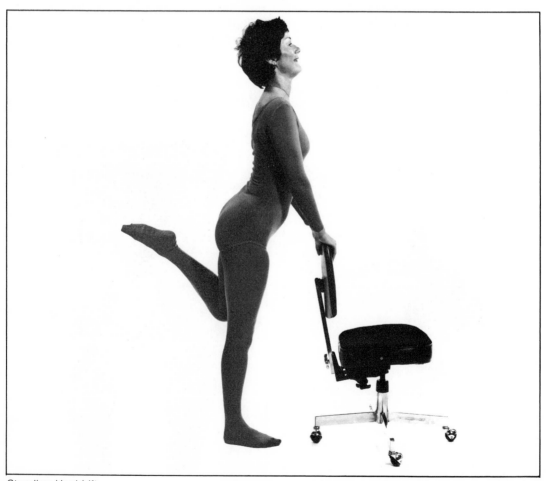

Standing Heel Lift

STANDING HEEL LIFT

Supporting yourself with your hands against a wall or chair, stand erect. Keeping knees together kick one leg back and up as high as you can. Keep the knee in place beside the opposite knee – all the motion is with the foot and lower leg. Return to starting position and repeat as fast as you can. Alternate legs each set.

Reps: 4x20 to 4x50   Rest: 15 sec.

 CROSS LEG PULL-IN

Lie face down on floor with ankles crossed. Keeping knees on floor, lift bottom leg up behind you as far as possible, resisting as hard as you can with the upper ankle. Return slowly to starting position, resisting strongly throughout. Then cross ankles in the opposite direction and repeat. Do not hold your breath.

Reps: 3x6 each leg to 3x10
Rest: 15 sec.

Knees

Pudgy, knobby, and straight knees are caused by lack of good muscle definition. Pudgy knees are usually compounded by fat deposits, principally on the inside of the upper knee, and at the back of the leg.

Recommended exercises include Half Squats, nos. 7 to 12, in Chapter 5.

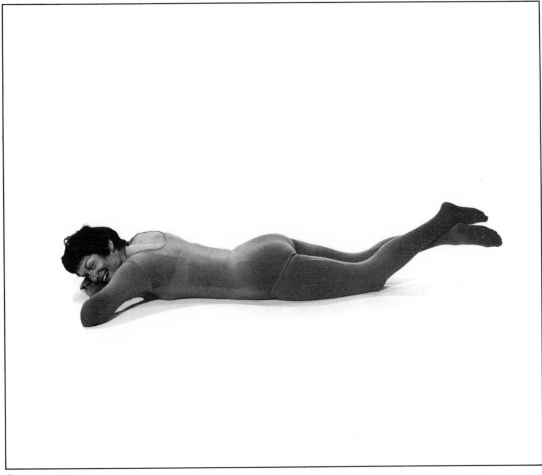

Cross Leg Pull-In

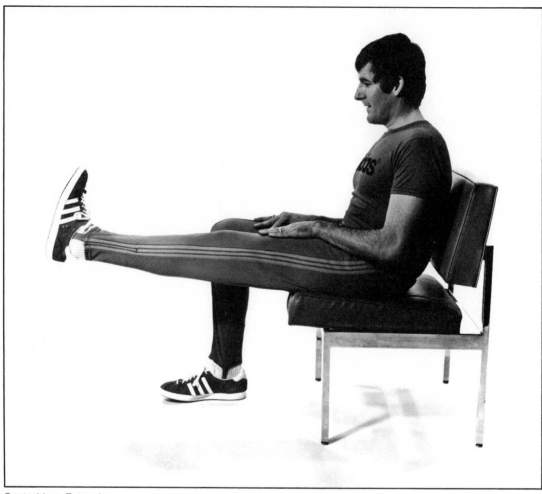

Seated Leg Extension

ex SEATED LEG EXTENSION

Sit on a chair, feet flat on floor. Extend one leg until straight. The movement is an *extension* of each leg rather than simply a swinging of the leg up and down. Alternate legs each set.

If your objective is to add contour to knobby or straight knees, use weighted boots or a substitute.

   Reps: 8x6   **Rest:** 15 secs.
   Add weight as able.

If your objective is to firm up flabby knees, instead of adding weights increase repetitions.

   Reps: 6x20 to 6x50   **Rest:** 15 sec.

Lower Legs

There is no real remedy for thick ankles. You can increase the contour of the calf muscles and of the muscles on the side and front of the leg so that the relative prominence of the ankle is decreased. Walk on tiptoe while holding weights in your hands, and walk on your heels. The more weight you can handle, the better the results. This and the following exercise will help remedy another problem with the lower leg – lack of contour in the calf area (''pipestem legs'').

In addition, try the Half Squats, nos. 7 to 12 in Chapter 5.

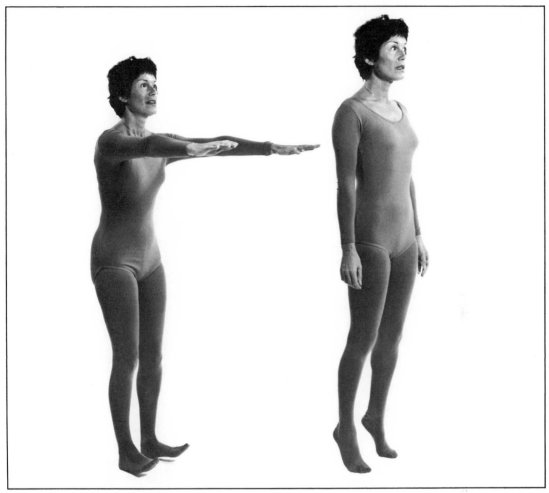

Toe-Heel Rock

 TOE-HEEL ROCK

Stand erect on tiptoe. Hold for 3 seconds, then rock slowly back onto heels and hold for 3 seconds. For added contour, you can increase resistance by holding something heavy across your shoulders (improvise with weight taped to a broomstick if you do not have a barbell).

Reps: 8x6   Add weights as able.
Rest: 15 sec.
To slim flabby calves, do not add weight but increase repetitions.

Reps: 3 x 20 to 3 x 50   **Rest:** 15 sec.

MIDSECTION

Abdomen

One of the first areas to lose the battle against gravity is the stomach. When the abdomen, burdened with extra fat, starts to sag, the internal organs descend with it. This may impair their function. Your posture will also suffer, and you will be prone to develop or aggravate low back problems. Girdles and other support garments are no real solution. They hide the symptom but do not cure the cause which is loss of muscle tone. The right solution is a "girdle" of strong, well-toned muscles.

Quite apart from the pleasing appearance of a flat stomach, these muscles are extremely important to your whole physical structure since they help to hold the pelvis in place. Many cases of low back pain can be traced to weak abdominals which have allowed the pelvis to tilt, placing excessive strain on the spinal column.

Many older persons starting on jogging campaigns have had to do special abdominal development in order to prevent low back pain from becoming a real problem.

A postural defect of the spine known as lordosis may be responsible for a certain amount of stomach prolapse, since it causes you to stand with the hips and pelvis forward. Check your posture to see if this is your problem, and refer to the section on lordosis in this chapter for remedial exercises.

Jack-knife exercises (nos. 24 to 28) in which the upper body and legs are brought together simultaneously are excellent for the abdominals. They give all the muscles a workout without throwing stress on the discs of the spine. Use the same progression system as suggested for squats, and remember that the exercises are listed in order of difficulty.

Exercises 20 to 23 are extremely valuable as well.

 HIGH STRETCH PULL-IN HOLD

Stand erect, feet comfortably apart. Reach up as high as you can, pulling your stomach in and up under the rib cage on the *exhale*. Hold 5 seconds. Inhale and relax.

This is a dual purpose exercise. Not only is it an excellent stomach flattener, but it also strengthens muscles which fight the downward drag of gravity, helping you to stand tall.

Reps: 10x5 sec. to 20x5
Rest: 10 sec.

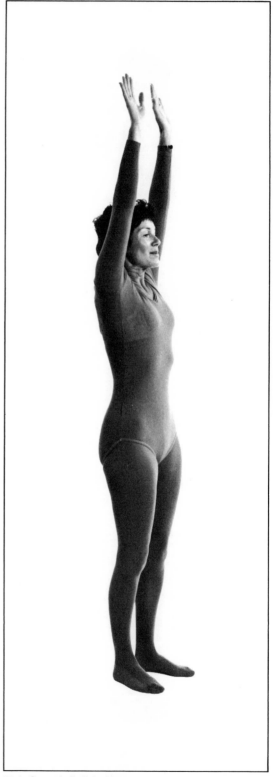

High Stretch Pull-In Hold

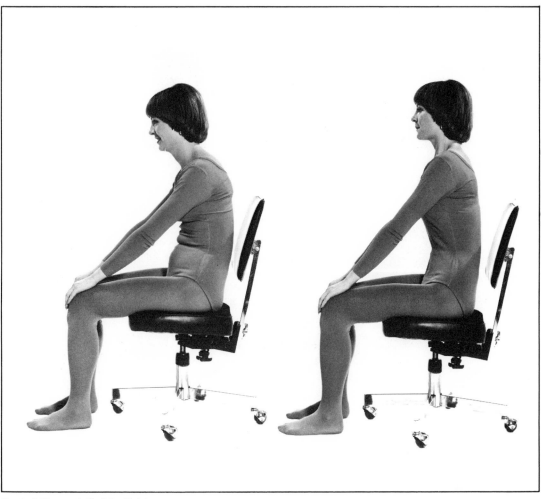

Seated Stomach Pull-In Hold

 SEATED STOMACH PULL-IN HOLD

Sit on the edge of a chair, feet flat on the floor, hands on knees. While *exhaling*, pull your stomach in and up as far as you can, pressing hard on your knees. Hold for 5 seconds. Inhale and relax. Rest 5 seconds and repeat.

This exercise firms up the stomach and arm muscles at the same time. You can do it anytime – while watching television, reading a book or sitting in your car waiting for the lights to change.

Reps: as many and as often as you can.

Buttocks

One of the most common of all figure faults is excess weight in the back of the upper legs, the seat, and the lower hip region. We spend so much of our time sitting that fat accumulates and the muscles start to sag.

Diet, which is an essential part of any campaign to tone up the buttock area, often fails to work satisfactorily. The muscles still sag.

The exercises listed here will help to remedy the problem, but to regain the youthful appearance you once had, additional activity may be necessary.

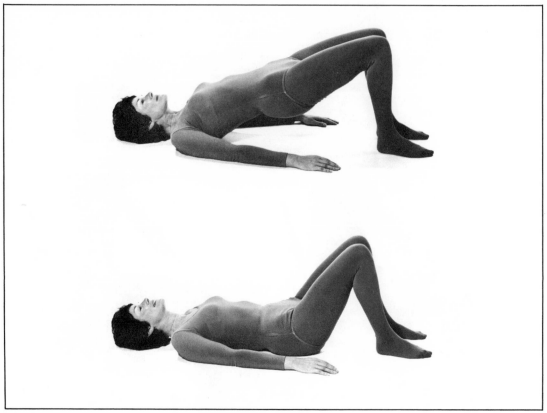

Hip Lift

Walking fast or running up and down stairs provide a good workout for this particular area. So does the Step Up (no. 16). Swimming, cross-country skiing and long stride walking or skating are other activities with particular benefits for the *gluteus maximus* muscles – the buttock muscles that do most of the work, and that sag the most noticeably if not sufficiently exercised.

 HIP LIFT

Lie on your back with knees bent, feet flat on floor, arms at sides, palms down. Tensing the buttocks, lift hips with an upward thrusting movement until body is in a straight line. Don't arch back. Relax buttocks and return to floor.

Reps: 3x8 to 3x20   **Rest:** 15 sec.

ex STRAIGHT LEG BACK LIFT

Lie on your stomach, legs straight, chin resting on hands. Lift one leg as high as you can, keeping the knee straight and the foot pointing straight down. (Turning the foot to one side decreases the load on certain key muscles.) Think of lifting the heel first. Alternate legs each set. Weights may be fastened to the feet for further resistance or an elastic belt may be looped around the ankles.

Reps: 8x10 to 8x20   **Rest:** 15 sec.

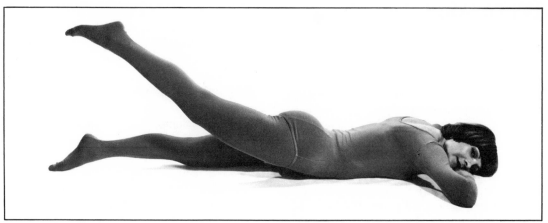

Straight Leg Back Lift

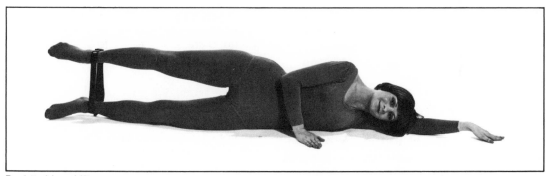

Resisted Leg Lift

Waist and Hips

Many hip-building or reducing exercises are unsuccessful because they do not load the muscles enough to bring about real change. Curves require muscles; if you're hoping to change the shape of your hips, you have to change the muscles. Resistance exercises are the only effective way to do this.

If your hips are flat and lacking in form, the leg lift exercise will build the appropriate muscles to provide curves in the right places. If they are too heavy, the same exercise will help to tighten up the muscles and make your hips and waist firmer.

As a bonus, this exercise also helps to improve the conformation of the abdomen, outer thighs, buttocks, and lower back. The tone and shape of the muscles in these areas also affect the appearance of your hips because the muscle system is closely linked.

That's why you should do all the midsection and leg exercises recommended in this section.

 RESISTED LEG LIFT

Lie on your left side with an elastic belt looped around your ankles. Lift right leg as high as possible, keeping knee straight and toes pointing forward. Hold for 5 seconds and return leg slowly to floor. Alternate sides each set.

If your objective is to add contour and form to your hips, use the strongest belt you can handle. If firming and reducing is your aim, use a light belt and double the number of reps.

Alternate positions: lying on your back (tones hips and front thighs), face-down (tones buttocks and back of thighs).

Reps: 4x8   **Rest:** 15 sec.

UPPER BODY

Everything from the waist up can be considered upper body, a neglected, abused portion of the human structure. It contains the lungs, heart, stomach, and other vital organs, is supported by the spine (which nature apparently never intended to be hoisted into an upright position), and is a platform for the head and arms.

Despite its importance, we give it less maintenance and care than we do our cars. We allow it to slump, we permit the muscles to get weak and out of tune, we overload it with fat, and we ignore its flexibility so that the lungs become cramped for "breathing room". Most of the attention we provide is cosmetic: covering up the bony parts, buttressing the sagging breasts, disguising the structural defects.

The result is a host of real problems which increase with age. They include such disorders of the spine as scoliosis, kyphosis and lordosis, sagging shoulders, and forward head; muscular weaknesses which prevent us from putting in a full working day without aches and pains in the neck and shoulders; and cramped living quarters for the stomach, liver, kidneys, and heart which are unable to function at full efficiency.

Let's look at some of the things we can do to repair this leaning tower of pizza.

Kyphosis

Kyphosis is a deviation of the spine resulting in a rounding of the upper back. Round shoulders and a forward head position always accompany kyphosis. Eventually, the large pectoral muscles in the chest, and the muscles lying between the ribs shorten. The flexibility of the rib cage becomes limited, and the total impression is one of hangdog depression and fatigue. The decreased expansion of the rib cage will ultimately affect breathing.

We can blame our life style for a lot of the difficulty. Sitting bent over a desk all day can lead to kyphosis. Instead of leaning forward at the hips, we invariably thrust the head forward and flex the entire spine in an effort to perform a task — writing, reading, typing — more easily.

Peering at television, driving cars, or bending over for long periods will also induce this postural slump. So will exceptionally heavy breasts, unless a brassiere with good support and wide shoulder straps is worn.

The first step in remedying the situation is to pay attention to the way you sit and stand. Lean from the hips, rather than thrusting the head forward. The accompanying exercises are designed to tone up the stretched muscles on the upper back and neck, and to stretch the shortened muscles of the chest. Also good are exercises 31 to 36, 40, 41, 46, and 59 in Chapter 5.

 HEAD PULL BACK HOLD

Stand or sit. Drop head until chin touches chest and clasp hands behind top of head. Now slowly move head up and back as far as possible, resisting strongly with your hands. When your head has gone as far back as you can move it, hold for a slow count of 5, maintaining resistance with the hands. Relax.

Reps: 6x5 sec.   Rest: 5 sec.

 ELBOWS BACK HOLD

Stand or sit erect, head tilted back slightly and stomach well in. Bend arms so forearms make a right angle and raise them to shoulder level with palms facing ahead. Now move arms back as far as possible, puffing out your chest. Keep your eyes straight ahead so that you do not change the position of your head. Hold for 10 seconds and relax. This will help to strengthen the back muscles and chest structure.

Reps: 10x10 sec.   Rest: 5 sec.

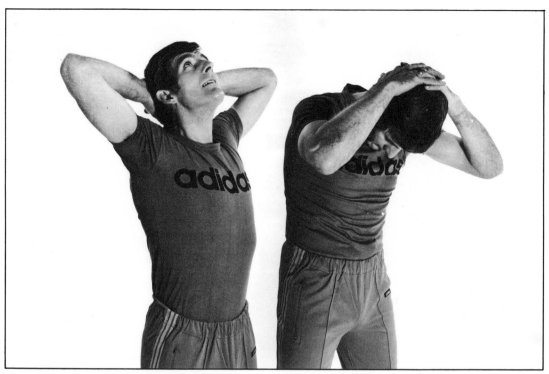

Head Pull Back Hold

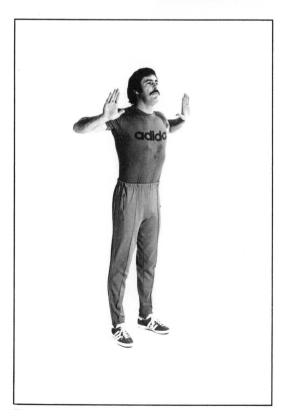

Elbows Back Hold

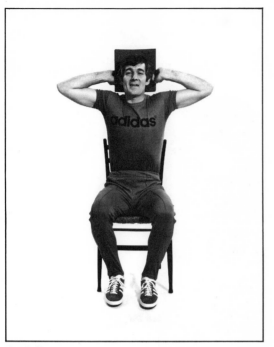

Book Press

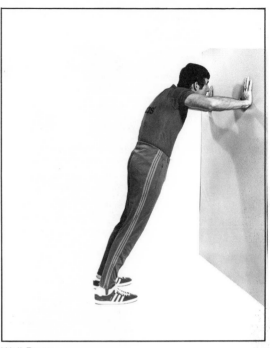

Wall Press

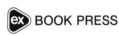 BOOK PRESS

With back well-supported in a high-backed chair, press a book hard against the back of your head. Keep head erect, eyes straight ahead, and resist the pressure of the book so that head remains in a stationary position. Hold for 10 seconds and relax. Breathe normally. This exercise helps to strengthen back and neck muscles.

Reps: 8x10 sec.　**Rest:** 10 sec.

Shoulder Blades

Prominent shoulder blades – sometimes called "wings" – are closely related to kyphosis and are caused by the same posture habits and occupational hazards. They too result in stretched muscles in the back and shortened ones in the chest, weakening the support of the upper body and throwing the head and shoulders forward.

After a time, the scapulae (shoulder blades) can be brought back into proper alignment only with difficulty. This is why it is valuable to catch the fault early; watch for signs of it in your children.

Exercise can do two things. It can tone up and strengthen the appropriate muscles to help you hold good posture, and it can build up the muscles of the back so that the shoulder blades are less apparent. Very often children have prominent wings simply because their backs are underdeveloped.

The following exercises as well as those listed for kyphosis are valuable in remedying this fault.

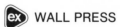 WALL PRESS

Place hands against wall at shoulder-height and shoulder-width apart with elbows bent at a 45 degree angle. Adjust distance of feet from wall for balance. Slowly push against the wall, exerting as much pressure as you can. Hold for 5 seconds and relax.

Reps: 8x5 sec.　**Rest:** 5 sec.

BENT ARM LATERAL PULL BACK

Place finger tips against back of neck. Keep head erect. Force elbows back as far as you can and hold for 5 seconds. Relax and return arms to sides.

Reps: 8x5 sec.   **Rest:** 5 sec.

STRAIGHT/BENT ARM PULL BACK

Raise straight arms in front to shoulder height, palms facing down, hands relaxed. Swing arms horizontally back behind body as far as they will go. Return to starting position. Repeat same movement, this time bending the elbows as arms swing back so that the hands move in beside the shoulders. Alternate straight/bent arm movements.

Reps: 2x10 to 2x20   **Rest:** 15 sec.

Scoliosis

Viewed from the side, the head, chest, and pelvic areas of a perfectly aligned body should be stacked one on top of the other so that a straight line would pass through the center of the ear, shoulder, hip, knee, and in front of the ankle. If one part of the body is out of place, the rest of the body must realign itself to compensate.

One problem which results from such a shift is kyphosis. A second one is scoliosis – a sideways curvature of the spine. This can be caused by one leg being shorter than the other, or by posture habits such as slumping the bodyweight over one hip when standing, or habitually lying on one side to read or watch television.

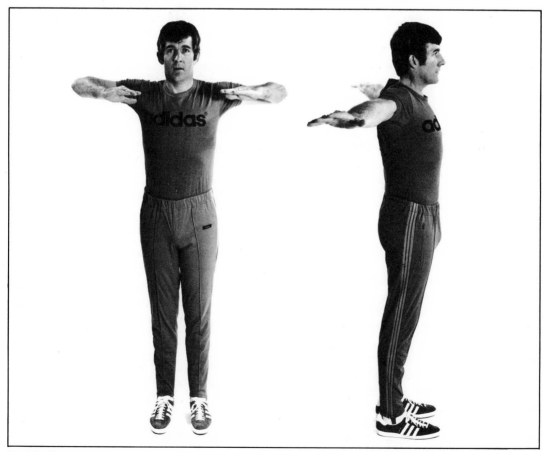

Straight/Bent Arm Pull Back

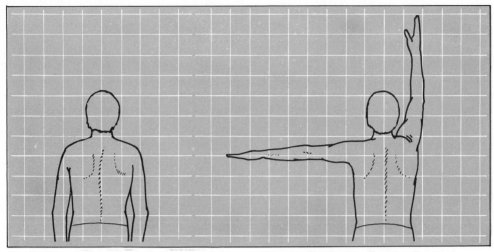

Scoliosis   Keynote Position to Test for Scoliosis

There are two forms of scoliosis: functional and structural. Left unattended, the first frequently deteriorates into the second, and this can create medical problems. For one thing, it cannot be cured, although further progression can be prevented through remedial exercises advised by a physician. Sometimes surgery is required.

The time to tackle scoliosis, then, is in the functional stage, and preferably early when it is easier to correct.

Check for scoliosis by standing with your back to a long mirror, and using a hand mirror to examine your spine for lateral curvature. A friend can do it for you. The important thing is to stand straight without turning the head.

THE KEYNOTE POSITION

If you think you detect a scoliosis, use what is called the "Keynote Position" to determine whether it is functional or structural. If your upper spine curves to the left, raise your right arm straight over your head (or vice versa). Lift the other arm out sideways to shoulder height. If the scoliosis disappears, it is functional; if it does not, it is probably structural, and a doctor should be consulted.

Assuming you have a functional scoliosis, you may find that it is caused by one leg

being shorter than the other. A lift in the shoe or on one heel will sometimes help. You should also concentrate on exercises which increase back and chest flexibility and which combat the lateral curving by stretching the muscles on the opposite side. Three of these are described here.

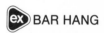 BAR HANG

This exercise requires a bar or some overhead structure you can use to get your feet off the ground. Grasp the bar with hands shoulder-width apart and hang from fully-extended arms as long as you can. Head should drop to chest. Rest until recovered.

Reps: 3 reps to 6 reps.

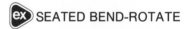 SEATED BEND-ROTATE

Sit in a chair with stomach in, chest high, and head erect. Clasp hands on top of head and bend over sideways as far as possible. Hold for 5 seconds. Now bend to other side and hold.

Next, rotate upper body to the right as far as you can. Hold for five seconds and repeat to the left.

Reps: 2x10 bends and 2x10 rotations. **Rest:** 15 sec.

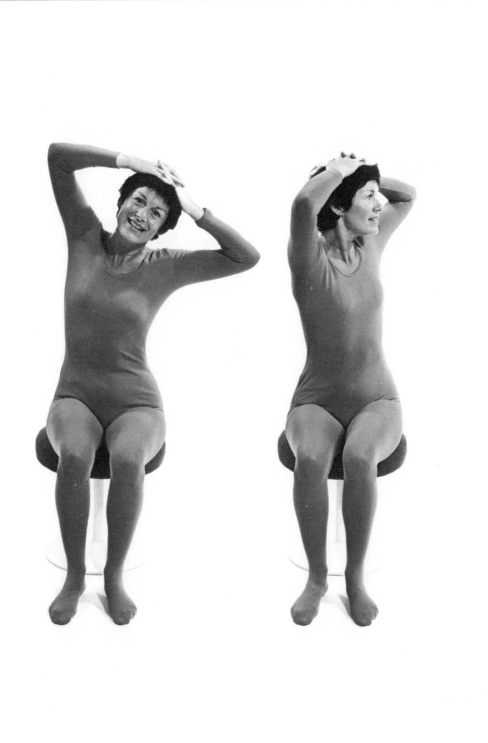

Seated Bend-Rotate

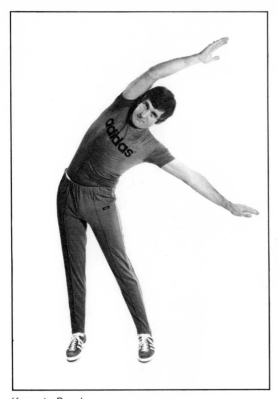

Keynote Bend

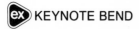 **KEYNOTE BEND**

Assume the keynote position described above to help you decide whether your scoliosis is structural or functional. Leading with the arm which is at shoulder height, bend over sideways as far as you can, hold for 5 seconds and return to the starting position. Repeat 10 times, switch arm position and repeat to the opposite side 5 times. Then switch arms again and do 10 more bends to the side with which you started.

Lordosis

Kyphosis, scoliosis, and finally lordosis – the Big Three of spinal abnormalities. Sometimes called swayback, lordosis is the exaggerated lower back curve which allows the pelvis and the abdomen to drop forward. It may be

responsible for slipped discs, and by compressing the openings between the vertebrae through which the spinal nerves pass may lead to low back pain.

Wearing high-heeled shoes and standing in one position aggravate swayback because of the attendant pressure on the nerves around the bottom of the spine. If you have to stand for a long period, find a low stool or a few books to use as a rest for one foot so that the hip joint is flexed. Change feet from time to time.

Pregnancy can aggravate a lordosis. The extra strain on the abdominal muscles tends to make them sag, and as the expectant mother tries to counter-balance herself the pelvis slips forward and the lower back curves in. That is why it is very important to do exercises which strengthen the abdominal muscles during pregnancy.

Sleeping habits are another aggravating factor in lordosis. Habitually sleeping on your stomach or back produces tensions which force the spine into a swayback position. Sleep on your side with the knees bent or, if you *must* sleep on your back, put a pillow under your knees.

Sitting in a chair with the hips higher than the knees is yet another culprit. The old-fashioned footstool did have a practical purpose. Take a look at your sitting posture when you're driving your car. Are your legs stretched out like a racing driver's to reach the pedals? Not so good. Adjust your seat so that it's slightly closer to the dash, raising your knees above hip level.

Mothers should watch their children for signs of a developing lordosis and take steps to correct it from the start. Children often try to emulate their parents, even to the extent of standing the same way. If you have an exaggerated curving-in of the lower back, and stand with your pelvis thrust forward and down, watch out that your child does not do the same. It could lead to back troubles later on.

A swayback that's been with you for many years may be difficult to correct – but not

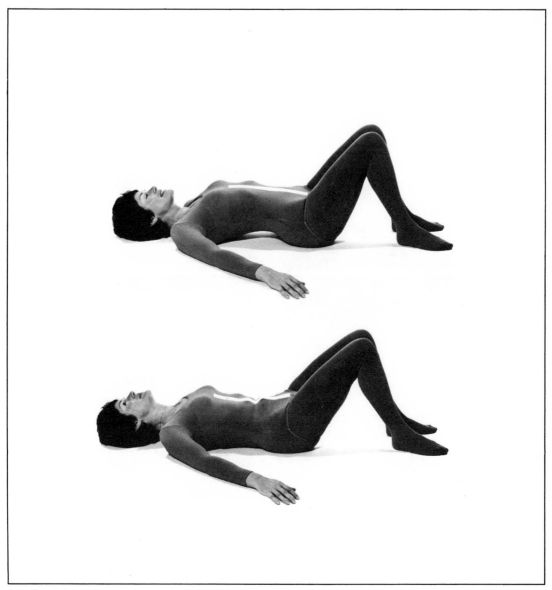

Low Back Press Down

impossible. Certainly exercises can do a lot to improve the situation, and can keep it from getting worse. If you're carrying extra weight on the stomach, get if off – this is one of the major causes of lordosis and if you haven't got the problem yet, you could be well along the road to acquiring it .

In addition to the drills suggested here, do the exercises for the abdominal area as well.

 LOW BACK PRESS DOWN

Lie on the floor with your knees well bent, arms at sides. Exhale and pull in your stomach as far as you can, at the same time pressing down with your lower back, trying to touch it to the floor. Hold for 5 seconds, relax for 5 seconds and repeat.

Reps: 2x10.   **Rest:** 15 sec.

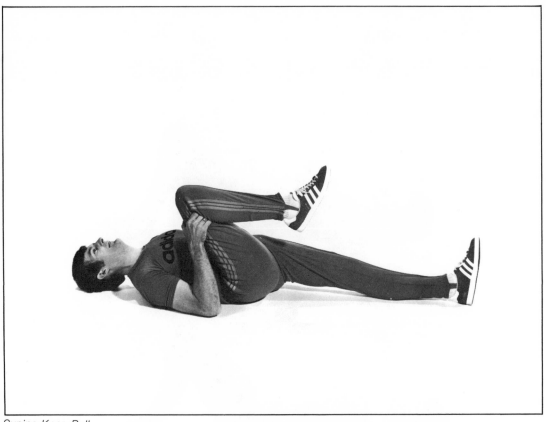

Supine Knee Pull

SUPINE KNEE PULL

Lie on back. Bend right leg and lift knee up toward the chest as far as you can. Clasp hands under knee and pull it steadily down toward the chest. Keep head and upper body on floor. Hold for 5 seconds, relax and repeat with other leg.

   Reps: 2x6.   **Rest:** 15 sec.

SEATED STOMACH PULL-IN

Sit erect, feet flat on floor, palms on top of legs just above knees. While exhaling, pull stomach in and up as far as you can. Relax while inhaling and repeat. This is not a holding movement but a continuous pulling in and up of the stomach.

   Reps: 2x8 to 2x30   **Rest:** 15 sec.

Chest

A manly chest was a symbol of male chauvinism long before the women's lib movement began. Similarly, the female bosom has had its own mystique. Braless or cantilevered, buttressed or undressed, the breast is as much a sociological symbol as it is a functional part of the human body.

   The breasts, which are composed principally of fatty and glandular tissue, cannot be made larger or smaller once they have reached maturity unless there are hormonal or weight changes, or through surgery. Nor can they be made firmer once they have started to sag. However, they can be made to *appear* larger and firmer by:

   1. Improved posture. If you slump, the breasts will appear to sag and will look smaller than they actually are.

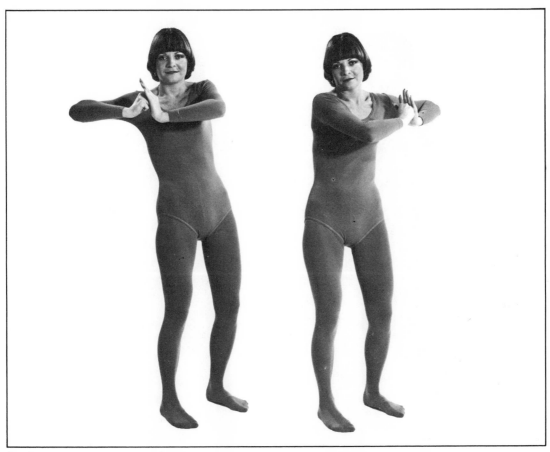

Fist Push Around

2. Development of the pectoral (front of the chest) muscles. This will lift the bosom and push it outwards. It will also help to support the weight of the breasts and prevent them from sagging.

By the way, doctors tend to disagree on the outcome of going braless. Many believe that after a period of time gravity will tend to drag the breasts downward. Once this occurs, even exercises will not cause them to bounce back.

The manly chest and womanly breasts have one thing in common in addition to their geographical location—both depend on muscle tissue and tone for maximum effect. The rippling pectorals which characterize Adonis on the beach may not be the average woman's goal, but strong chest development is the best insurance that her breasts will remain firm and youthful as the years go by. The exercises required for development in this area are the same for both sexes. As well as exercises 37 and 38 in the Bank, try the following:

 FIST PUSH AROUND

Make a fist. Cup it in the palm of other hand at side of body. Exert strong pressure against palm with fist and "push" across the front of the chest. Resist with the palm of the cupped hand. Keep shoulders low and chest high. Change hand position and push back the other way. Do not hold your breath.

Reps: 2x6 to 2x8   **Rest:** 15 sec.

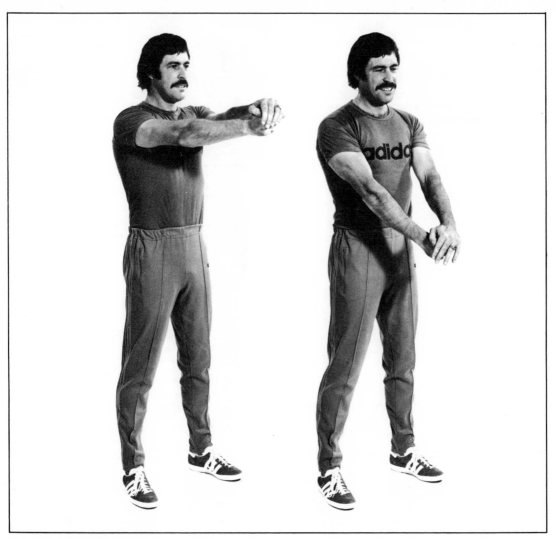

Resistance Press Down

 RESISTANCE PRESS DOWN

Extend both arms. Make a fist with the right hand and place left palm over it. Press down with the upper hand, resisting with the fist. Keep chest high and force the shoulders down. Hold for 5 seconds, relax, switch hands and repeat. Breathe normally.

Rep: 2x6 to 2x12   **Rest:** 15 sec.

Shoulders

The collarbones (clavicles) are slender S-shaped bones which hold the arms up and slightly away from the trunk, and transmit forces from the arms to the trunk. They also give support to the shoulder joints, and have important muscle attachments.

All that's been said about slump, kyphosis and other upper body problems applies here.

The same posture habits which throw the shoulders too far forward also create collarbones that protrude. In addition, people who are thin and lack development will display unattractive hollows and prominent bones at the bottom of the throat.

The muscles directly involved include the groups at the base of the neck, the deltoids (anterior shoulder muscles), the pectoralis major (the chest muscles), and the trapezius muscles of the back.

Fortunately, all these muscles respond readily to exercise. The exercises listed here (and exercises 31 to 36 in Chapter 5) will help you fill out those hollow spots quite quickly as well as making it easier to maintain good posture. In addition, you should do the exercises suggested earlier for kyphosis, the shoulder blades, and the bosom. Swimming is an excellent activity for strengthening and toning up the muscles of the shoulder girdle, particularly a vigorous crawl stroke with lots of arm action.

 FORWARD ARM LIFT

Stand erect holding a heavy book in front of your thighs. Keeping arms straight, slowly lift the book over your head, exhaling at the same time. Return slowly to starting position while inhaling. If you have barbells, build up to 3 or 4 pounds.

Rep: 3x8 to 3x30 **Rest:** 15 sec.

 LATERAL ARM LIFT

Hold books or light barbells at sides with arms straight. Slowly raise them out to the side and overhead as high as possible. Return slowly to starting position. Add weight as able.

Rep: 3x8 to 3x20 **Rest:** 15 sec.

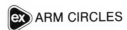 **ARM CIRCLES**

Using books or other resistance, extend arms to sides at shoulder height and make a plate-size circle. Alternate clockwise and anti-clockwise circles after every 5 reps. This exercise can be done with hands extended forward at eye level. Gradually increase weight (resistance) as able.

Rep: 2x10 to 2x30 **Rest:** 15 sec.

Neck

The adult head accounts for one seventeenth of the entire body weight. Obviously, a strong, well-positioned neck is essential if the head's to be held high and proud. Gravity is the enemy again. Year after year it tries to drag the head forward and down. If we let our posture go, we wind up with a double chin and the deep sag lines in the neck which indicate advancing years.

What about your posture? Do you like to slump in an easy chair with your buttocks on the front edge and your spine curved against the back? Do you lie in bed reading with several pillows propping up your head? Do you stand with your weight on your heels? What about your upper body when you're sitting at a desk or sewing machine? Is the head forward and the back rounded?

All these habits contribute to a double chin and sagging neck muscles.

The first step then, is to concentrate on your posture habits. When you stand, stand with your weight on the balls of your feet, the shoulder blades back and down, the chin level and somewhat forward. Sit erect. Check your posture when you're sitting at a desk; you'll suffer far less tension in the neck and shoulder muscles and those across the back if your carriage is upright and the head is balanced. Slumping forward gives the muscles extra work to do to keep the head from dropping down on your chest.

The second step is to check your nutrition. If you're overweight, chances are some of the flab is going to collect under your chin.

Finally, exercises. Fortunately, the neck muscles are among the most easily developed of the entire body. The following exercises will quickly strengthen and tone up muscles which are weak and flabby, and help you regain a more youthful neck-line. In conjunction with these, you should include the exercises for the shoulders, upper back, chest, and shoulder blades, all of which help to hold your body in good postural alignment.

 HEAD CIRCLING

Sit or stand erect. Without slumping, let the head fall forward until your chin touches your chest. Now move the head slowly in a wide circle to the right until you are back at your starting position. Reverse and make a big circle to the left.

Reps: 2x4 to 2x6   **Rest:** 15 sec.

 RESISTANCE DRILL

This is a three-stage exercise.

1. With the head tilted well back, press fingertips of both hands against your forehead. Move head forward and down, providing moderate resistance with your hands. Relax, return to sitting position and repeat 3 times.

2. Tilt head forward so that the chin is on chest. Place fingers on back of head. Now lift head up and back as far as possible, resisting moderately with hands. Relax, return to starting position and repeat 3 times.

3. Tilt head to right, trying to touch your ear to your shoulder. Place fingers of left hand against left temple and move your head up and over toward left shoulder, resisting with hand. Repeat to opposite side. Do 3 reps each side.

These stages can be repeated 3 or 4 times. If you want a slimming effect use mild resistance and increased repetitions. If you are looking for fullness and improved neck development, gradually increase the degree of resistance.

 THE BULLDOG

Move head well back with chin up. Now stick your chin out trying to force the lower jaw forward as far as you can. Hold maximum stretch for 3 seconds, then relax and repeat.

Reps: 2x6 to 2x10   **Rest:** 15 sec.

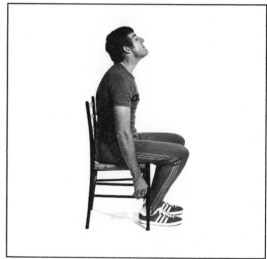

The Bulldog

Arms

Many people, unless they are heavily involved in sports or jobs which demand upper body strength, lack good development of the muscles in their arms. For the average city dweller there just aren't enough activities requiring arm strength to ensure proper growth of the biceps, triceps, and flexors.

Women have particular problems. Society decrees that a woman shall not participate in activities which either demand or create muscles, particularly in the arms. She may play tennis, but not football; she may do housework, but is expected to call for male help when heavy lifting is required; she plants the flowers while husband does the digging.

The old rules are vanishing, of course, and many people always did ignore them. But one of the byproducts of this system is arms which are underdeveloped and hence not as attractive as they might be. The wrists may be slender — but so are the forearms, and the wrists look less slender by contrast, not to mention their being unequal to activities which demand wrist strength. The triceps muscles on the bottom of the upper arms start to sag slightly as the years go by and fat accumulates, even though mother is expected to do the housework and carry the groceries. That kind of lifting and carrying activity is good for the biceps, but doesn't do much for the triceps.

Many older persons — and even some very young ones — suffer from lack of tone and firmness of the triceps muscle. This is a relatively easy fault to put right, even when you are well into your 50s and 60s. Thin forearms are more difficult — but not impossible. Filling out the arms will improve the appearance of the wrists by reducing the prominence of the ends of the bones and will increase their strength so that you can do everyday tasks much more easily.

Fairly heavy exercise is required to "gather" and strengthen the muscles, while high repetitions will condition them and help get rid of fat.

Swimming is a good build-up activity for the arm muscles, particularly the crawl stroke with its pressing-down action involving the triceps.

 KNEE PRESS DOWN

Sit erect, feet flat on floor, hands on knees. Keeping arms straight, press down on the knees as hard as you can for 5 seconds. Relax for 5 seconds, then repeat.

Reps: 6 reps to 12 reps.

 PUSH-PULL

Raise hands to chin level. Make a fist with your right hand and cup it in the palm of the left hand. Using moderate resistance from your left arm, press it out away from you until arms are fully extended. Then pull the left arm back to the starting position, resisting with the right. Change hands and repeat. Breathe normally.

Reps: 3x6 to 3x12   **Rest:** 15 sec.

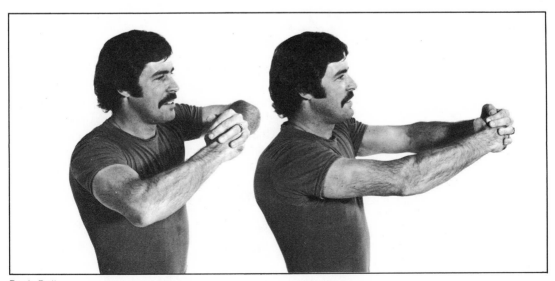

Push-Pull

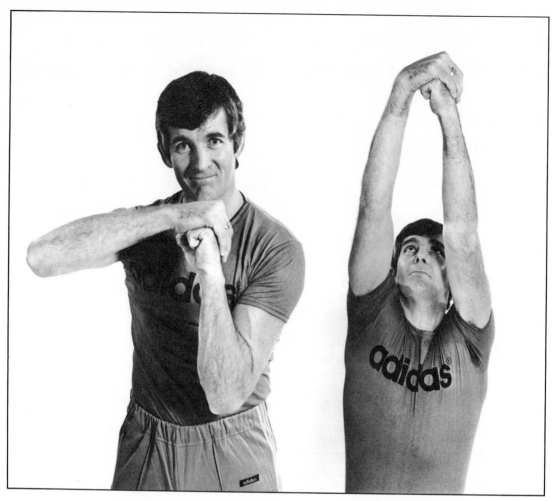

Resisted Arm Lift

ⓔⓧ RESISTED ARM LIFT

Make a fist with one hand and cup the other palm over it opposite your chin. Resisting with the palm, extend arms overhead. Return to starting position, resisting with bottom hand. Change hands and repeat. Start with moderate resistance and build to maximum resistance.

Reps: 3x4 to 3x8   **Rest:** 15 sec.

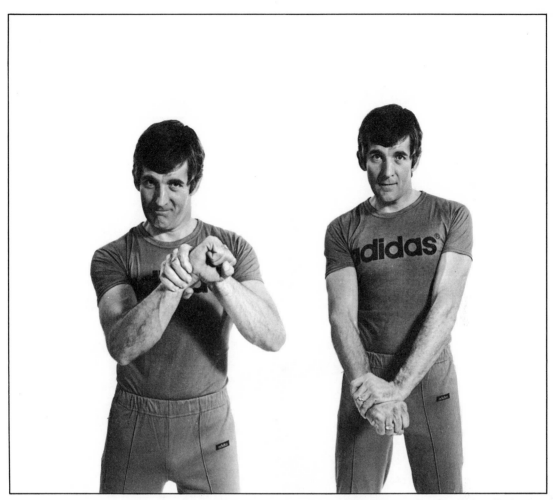

Single Arm Resistance

 SINGLE ARM RESISTANCE

Extend right arm down in front of the body. Bend left arm and grasp right wrist. Flex right arm and bring the wrist up toward the opposite shoulder, resisting throughout with the left arm. Return to starting position resisting with the right arm. Change hands and repeat. Build resistance from moderate to maximum.

Reps: 3x4 to 3x8   **Rest:** 15 sec.

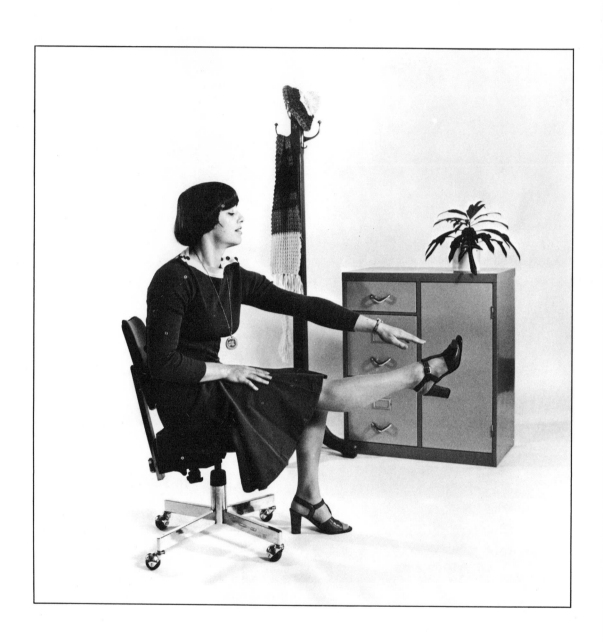

Fitness
and
Daily Living

7 Nutrition

HEALTHY EATING HABITS

Good nutrition is the art of eating wisely. But there's more to it than getting enough of the right vitamins, minerals, and other nutrients. You should get them in the right proportions, your calorie intake should be appropriate for the weight you want to maintain, and you should keep to a minimum those food elements – animal fats and refined sugar, for example – which can be harmful in excessive quantities.

By eating a lot, many people get all the vitamins and minerals they need, but they also become too fat. This makes them candidates for certain diseases, particularly those relating to the heart and cardiovascular system. Others who also overeat still do not get all the necessary food elements. Their diets are not only out of balance, they are deficient, even though these individuals may be seriously overweight.

The problem is insidious. The individual may appear perfectly healthy, yet the legacy of his deficiencies is there; it will make itself felt as he gets older. As he passes middle age, he may begin to suffer from ailments directly related to careless and carefree eating when young.

Surveys have exposed certain eating patterns in industrialized countries – overindulgence in junk foods, and overreliance on instant dinners at the expense of green vegetables and salads. The problem appears to be based more on ignorance or carelessness than on socioeconomic factors. Those in lower-income brackets often eat more wisely than those who can afford to indulge their appetite for exotic foods.

The following is a list of the most likely imbalances in the diet of the average person:

1. Too much animal fat. This appears to be the greatest single dietary indiscretion. Not only does it contribute to obesity, but it has been strongly linked to atherosclerosis (fatty build up in the blood vessels) and other circulatory problems.

2. Too much refined sugar. Second in line, a strong challenger to become number one. Combined with too little physical activity, it creates probably the most hazardous of all dietary problems. It is linked with cholesterol build up, with obesity, with diabetes and dental caries.

3. Too little B-complex. Whole grain breads and cereals, some meats, turnips, and natural supplements such as wheat germ contain high concentrations of the B-complex

vitamins. They are important in the utilization of carbohydrates for energy, in the health of the nervous system, and in regulating heart function. Many people rely on pills to provide these vitamins, but natural foods are far better. Bread used to be an important source; nowadays the germ of the wheat is absent, except in 100 per cent whole-wheat bread, and with it most of the B-complex series. Sixty per cent whole wheat is inadequate, because the missing 40 per cent is the germ.

4. Too few fresh vegetables. Vegetables, especially the green ones, provide many of the important minerals required by the body. Canned vegetables cannot compare with those that are freshly prepared or, better yet, can be eaten raw. Cooking tends to destroy many vitamins and minerals.

5. Not enough calcium. Milk and cheese are the major sources. Don't let worry about weight and too much animal fat steer you away from these items. Make an effort to adjust to the taste and texture of skim milk and skim-milk products, including low-fat cheese. It will be a valuable move.

6. Insufficient variety of protein. Meat is a good source of the so-called complete proteins, but also contains the highly suspect saturated fatty acids. Other valuable sources of protein which should be staple parts of the diet are: beans, nuts, soybeans, lentils, whole-wheat products, and rice.

7. Not enough potassium. Many people get very little of this chief intracellular mineral which is vital to virtually all the life-sustaining processes and the energy structure. Bananas and potatoes are excellent sources.

8. Not enough vitamin C. Vitamin C is not stored in the body and must be replenished daily, yet many people have only intermittent intake of this vitamin which is found in citrus fruits and tomatoes. Its role in fighting off infections has been well documented. It also is related to the health of the arterial system and the function of the adrenal glands.

The Many Faces of Protein

About 20 per cent of the food we eat should consist of protein, which contains the 22 amino acids that are vital to the growth, maintenance, and repair of body cells. The 8 so-called "essential" amino acids are those the body cannot manufacture for itself.

Proteins found in meat and other animal sources such as eggs, cheese, and milk, are known as "complete" proteins because they contain all the essential amino acids. Those found in vegetables are generally considered incomplete, because one or more of these acids may be missing or present in very small quantities. Soybeans are one of the few vegetable sources of complete proteins.

Should we then get all our protein from meat, fish, eggs, and ignore the vegetable sources: beans, wheat, peas, soybeans, lentils, nuts, corn, rye, and yeast? Not so. Meat sources have a serious drawback in that they tend to be very high in cholesterol and fats which are closely linked with certain heart-circulatory disorders, including arteriosclerosis (hardening of the arteries).

In addition to being relatively free of saturated fats, vegetable sources of protein are high in certain vitamins and minerals not found in meat, and those containing Vitamins C and E are valuable for anyone worried about possible cholesterol build up.

Fortunately, even small amounts of a complete protein can fulfill a vegetable protein and make it complete. However, vegetarians, or those on a high-vegetable diet, should make sure to get plenty of variety. In this way, a protein source that is low in a particular amino acid will be counterbalanced by one that has an adequate amount of it.

In their book, *Nutrition and Physical Fitness*, L. Jean Bogert, George M. Briggs and Doris Calloway,[1] warn that a totally vegetarian diet makes it difficult to obtain certain nutrients, especially calcium, iron, fat-soluble vitamins such as A, D, E and K, and complete proteins. They recommend including some foods of animal origin.

For example, here is their estimate of the total equivalent non-meat foods you would have to eat in order to obtain the complete protein value contained in just one 2½ oz. serving of meat: 1½ cups of cooked dried beans or peas, 1 cup of cooked soybeans, 3 oz. of cheese, 3 tablespoons of peanut butter, ¾ cup of cottage cheese, 2½ glasses of milk.

If you're thinking about shifting to a smaller proportion of meat in your diet, or perhaps eliminating it altogether, following is a list of some good sources of vegetable protein. Remember to eat a variety of them in order to obtain all the necessary amino acids.

FOOD SOURCE	GRAMS TOTAL PROTEIN	CALORIES
Oatmeal (1 cup cooked)	5.4	148
Rice (1 cup dry white, milled)	14.5	692
Macaroni (1 cup dry, enriched)	13.7	405
Wheat germ (3-1/2 oz. commercial)	26.6	363
Peanuts (3-1/2 oz. roasted)	26.5	572
Peanut butter (1 cup)	67.3	1486
Dried beans (1/2 cup white)	22.3	340
Lima beans (5/8 cup dried)	20.4	345
Soybeans (1/2 cup dried)	34.1	403
Black bean soup (1 can condensed)	15.3	261
Green pea soup (1 can condensed)	16.6	339
Canned beans (1/2 cup)	7.9	150
Lentils (1/2 cup split, dry)	24.7	340
Potato (2-1/2 in. diameter, baked)	3.9	139
Potato (3-1/2 oz. dehydrated)	7.2	364
Whole wheat bread (1 slice)	2.4	56

Vitamin Supplementation

Vitamin and mineral supplementation is a controversial subject. Many people believe in it and take vitamin pills as a matter of course. Doctors say it isn't necessary — except for certain medical conditions — if the individual has "a good, balanced diet". But, a $2.5 million Nutrition Canada study which began in 1969 found that millions of Canadians were suffering from some form of malnutrition because they didn't eat properly, and 20 per cent of the people participating in the study had to be referred to doctors for treatment of medical problems arising from dietary deficiencies.

Does this mean that we should all be relying on pills to guarantee good nutrition? Dr. Zachary Sabry, the coordinator of the survey, doesn't believe this is a good idea. For one thing, most people don't know exactly what's missing from their diet. Vitamins often work properly only in conjunction with other vitamins and minerals. Dr. Sabry claims that there is no complete supplement on the market, despite the growing rows of vitamin and mineral pills in the drug stores.

One of the problems is that prepared foods often lose certain vital elements en route from field to you. Dr. Sabry says industry hasn't taken sufficient initiative in food enrichment to guarantee that you're getting what you *think* you're getting from your meals.

Then there are the junk foods. They're a short-cut meal for many working mothers; they are dispensed universally, even in schools, but they contain little nutrition. Millions of people, particularly growing youngsters, eat far too much of them. It's hard to sell good nutrition to the average young person.

Unless you're absolutely certain your nutrition pattern adheres to the "good, balanced diet" formula, some form of general-purpose supplementation is probably a good idea, particularly for athletes and active, growing youngsters. If in doubt, consult your family physician for specific recommendations.

Here are the principal vitamins and minerals and their areas of influence:

Vitamin A: Growth, vision, maintenance of tissue, development of teeth and health of skin, respiratory passages, digestive and urinary tracts.
  Good sources: Liver, fish liver oils, milk and milk products, egg yolk, spinach, broccoli, beans, carrots, lettuce, apricots, and peaches.

Vitamin B Complex: Release of energy from carbohydrate foods, normal red blood cell synthesis, aerobic metabolism of cells, maintenance of a healthy nervous system. Essential to many functions of the body.
  Good sources: Milk, yeast, liver, kidneys, fish, eggs, vegetables, lean meat, fresh fruits.

Vitamin C: Health of adrenal glands, defence against infection and stress, blood building, blood vessel elasticity, connective tissue, dispersal of fatigue acids, healing of tissues.
  Good sources: Citrus fruits, tomatoes, potatoes cooked in their jackets.

Vitamin D: Bone development. Important during growth years and pregnancy, limited need by adults.
  Good sources: Sunlight, fish liver oils, fortified milk.

Vitamin E: Improved capillarization and circulation, utilization of oxygen. Antagonist to cholesterol in blood, and a physiological compensator during metabolic stress.
  Good sources: Wheat germ, 100 per cent whole-wheat bread.

Iron: Manufacture of hemoglobin, the oxygen transport system. Lack of iron will contribute to fatigue and detract from physical performance, particularly endurance.
  Good sources: Meat, especially liver, eggs, leafy green vegetables, whole-grain cereals, molasses, dried fruits.

Calcium: Development of bones and teeth, coagulation of blood, passage of fluids through cell walls, action of enzymes, heart function, maintenance of muscles, and nerve sensitivity.
  Good sources: Milk, cheese, leafy green vegetables, and nuts.

Magnesium: Utilization of calcium, phosphorus and many important vitamins including B complex, C, and E. Involved in many essential metabolic processes, particularly carbohydrates and amino acids (proteins). Required for proper functioning of nerves and muscles, including those of the heart.
  Good sources: Fresh green vegetables, apples, corn, nuts, soybeans, and unmilled wheat germ.

Sodium: Chloride and sodium are principal minerals in blood plasma and extra-cellular fluids, and are dominant in the metabolism of body water. Body processes take place in salt solutions.
  Good sources: Salt, well-balanced diet.

Iodine: Function of thyroid gland.
  Good sources: Sea foods, iodized salt.

Fluoride: Resistance to tooth decay, particularly in the young.
> *Good sources:* Water containing fluoride, either naturally or by addition.

Copper: Manufacture of hemoglobin.
> *Good sources:* A well-balanced diet.

Phosphate: Maintaining the processes of most body cells, calcium function, and the metabolism of fat and carbohydrates.
> *Good sources:* milk, leafy green vegetables, nuts.

Potassium: The chief intracellular mineral, vital to virtually all the life-sustaining processes of body tissue; important in the energy-burning process and recovery from fatigue.
> *Good sources:* A well-balanced diet, potatoes, whole grains, dried fruits, bananas and nuts.

Dead Calories

Dead calories are exactly what the name implies – calories with no nutritive value. Most people eat far too many of them. Refined sugar which is a carbohydrate with most of the nutritive value removed is the major culprit. The average North American eats 100 lbs. of sugar every year – a total of some 178,000 calories.

In addition to the sugar you spoon into your tea or coffee, or on top of your cereal, refined sugar is found in hundreds of other food items: soups, prepared rice, baked beans, butter, mustard, catsup, crackers, many medicines, tinned vegetables, peanut butter, prepared cereals, candy, chocolate, soft drinks. The list goes on and on.

Our body's primary source of energy is carbohydrates. Sugars are just one of them; the others are starches and cellulose. In addition to producing calories for energy, they help to regulate protein and fat metabolism. Valuable natural sources include: cane sugar, honey, maple syrup, jams, jellies, fruits, and milk and malt sugar; plus such starchy foods as bread, flour, cereals, potatoes, milk, rice, most vegetables, cakes, and corn starch, all of which contain other nutritional elements.

The average person 80 years ago ate 28 per cent more carbohydrates than we do today. But our consumption of cereals has dropped 60 per cent and that of potatoes 50 per cent, while refined sugar consumption has gone up 130 per cent. This represents a significant shift toward dead calories.

One reason is the growth of the canned food industry where sugar is used not only to enhance flavor but as a preservative. Many cereals and other prepared products are touted in advertising as excellent sources of quick energy. However, they are not necessarily the *best* sources.

The trouble with quick energy sources is that the energy is soon lost, since the rush of insulin into the bloodstream reduces the glucose level very fast. Glucose is the primary energy source and is also obtained from starches, proteins, and fat. Proteins and starches are the best source of glucose since it is released more slowly and does not cause a sudden reaction from the body to get rid of the excess. The effect is slower, but longer lasting.

Some investigations have linked sugar with raised serum cholesterol and triglyceride levels, and diets high in cholesterol are usually high in sugar as well.

There are two more factors to consider. High sugar intake leads to dental caries, and reduces the quantities of more nutritious foods that we can eat. Next time you feel the urge for a chocolate bar, a soft drink, or a pastry snack, think again. Isn't there something else you'd rather have?

The Cholesterol Monster

Cholesterol is a constituent of almost all the body's cellular membranes and is vital to the production of certain hormones. We absorb it from our food, and the body synthesizes a certain amount from carbohydrates, proteins, and fats. In company with fats (known as lipids), triglycerides, phospholipids, and proteins, it contributes to coronary heart disease.

Many doctors are not convinced that eliminating cholesterol-containing foods from our diet is *the* answer to this problem. Research shows that some people with high-cholesterol diets are still relatively free of such symptoms as atherosclerosis (clogging) of the arteries, and have surprisingly low cholesterol levels in their blood. Regular physical activity, keeping weight levels down, and sufficient Vitamin C seem to play a role in this phenomenon.

Dr. Frederick J. Stare, head of the Department of Nutrition at Harvard University feels that it's not the cholesterol intake that hurts the heart, but letting cholesterol build up. Physical activity burns it up.

However, this doesn't mean that you should disregard what you eat. Large amounts of fat in the diet, particularly of saturated fat such as that found in fatty meats, lard, butter, and certain oils, stimulates the body's cholesterol production. But unsaturated and polyunsaturated fats – primarily vegetable fats such as corn oil which are usually liquid at room temperature – are active in reducing blood cholesterol.

The Intersociety Commission for Heart Diseases suggested that the average person should get no more than 300 milligrams of cholesterol per day – slightly more than is found in the yolk of one egg. As a matter of fact, the American Heart Association recommends that no more than three egg yolks should be eaten in a week by the average person. (This includes egg yolks used in cooking.) Other foods to watch are various organs (brain, liver, kidneys), shellfish, butter, lard, marbled-fat meats (including hamburger), and some luncheon meats.

Serum cholesterol levels are now measured as part of most medical checkups. Those with cholesterol levels approaching the danger line should follow their doctor's advice. Regular

exercise and staying slim appear to be the best defences against the cholesterol monster.

Keeping Your Bones Healthy

Elsewhere in this book we've looked at the effects of regular exercise in keeping the bones healthy and preventing a progressive disease known as osteoporosis – porous, brittle bones. Surveys show that many older people suffer from this problem, particularly women for whom after menopause the incidence may be as high as one in four.

There are three main causes: lack of exercise, hormone imbalance, and calcium deficiency.

Studies show a relatively low incidence of bone disease in countries where the average diet is rich in calcium foods – milk, cheese, and other dairy products, green leafy vegetables, nuts, sesame seeds, soybeans, molasses, and figs.

Vitamin D (found in sunshine, liver, eggs, salmon, sardines, and added to milk) also plays an important role in bone formation for it controls the release of phosphorus so that it can combine with calcium to form bone tissue. Adults normally obtain sufficient Vitamin D for health, but in growing children it may be necessary to provide such supplements as cod liver oil capsules.

Feeding the Family Athlete

What should athletes eat? There are almost as many theories as there are athletes and coaches. Medical science will allow itself few positive statements beyond "a good, balanced diet", since the exact effects of nutrition are difficult to study under a microscope. Hockey is just moving out of the "big steak before a game" era which disappeared in most other sports many years ago. (A big steak does nothing for the about-to-be-active athlete except sit in his stomach like a lead weight.) Swedish physiologist Dr.

Per-Olof Astrand has found ways to increase endurance through special carbohydrate feeding in the 10 days prior to an event, and iron-curtain countries are doing intensive studies of athletic nutrition.

There are some fundamental principles which all athletes should observe, and the "kitchen coach" is well advised to be aware of them. Nutrition plays a major role in helping the highly competitive athlete to combat physiological stress. What he or she eats and drinks on a regular basis will have a profound influence on physical capacity to sustain a hard training and competitive program throughout the year.

Let's take a look at the athlete's overall nutrition pattern: the pre-practice or pre-competition meal; the post-practice and post-game meal.

General Nutrition: An active athlete, particularly one involved in sports demanding high endurance, will need far more calories than the average person, perhaps as high as 6,000 per day. Exactly how many calories should be determined by keeping a close check on weight. If the athlete is lean – and most athletes are these days – the weight should not fluctuate much from day to day. There may be as much as 10 pounds difference after a practice or game, but that is fluid loss and is quickly replenished with liquids. If the mature athlete is gaining weight steadily, and is not on a bulk-building weight-training program, then the number of calories should be reduced. The opposite applies if the athlete is losing weight and is lean to start with.

The athlete must have adequate amounts of all the vitamins, minerals, and trace elements the body demands. A daily balanced diet should include: protein (meat, poultry, fish, whole-grain breads and cereals, milk, cheese, nuts); high vitamin/mineral foods (green salads and vegetables generally); fresh fruits (especially citrus fruits). Recommended proportions are: 40 per cent protein, 40 per cent starches/carbohydrates, 20 per cent fats (principally unsaturated vegetable fats – use vegetable oils in frying, roasting, salads).

If muscle building is required, or if the sport places high demands on muscle/strength work, increase the protein intake by 10 per cent. If it's a high-endurance activity (distance running, swimming, cross-country skiing), boost the starch/carbohydrate ratio and the citrus fruits. The latter help to keep the athlete's alkaline reserve high to combat fatigue acids.

Pre-competition Meal: Eat 2 or 3 hours before the event. Keep protein content low since it is not digested quickly. The meal should be high in calories (carbohydrate foods) but low in bulk, and free from condiments, spices, and fatty or fibrous foods. Include lots of citrus fruit and juices which leave an alkaline residue after digestion.

On the other hand, world records have been broken half an hour after a meal of hamburgers, potato chips, and coca cola; so, if the athlete wants a steak and has no stomach problems, he or she is probably better off eating it than feeling deprived. But do try for good pre-game nutrition whenever possible.

Post-Competition and Practice Replenishment: This is an important but often overlooked factor. The hard-working athlete uses up a number of salts, minerals, and "fuel" elements which need to be replenished to keep the machinery in good order. The meal should be a mixed one, with emphasis on carbohydrates, citrus fruits and fluids. Provide an extra sprinkling of salt if he or she has been perspiring heavily. It should also be highly digestible. Postpone it until the athlete is rested. If he or she doesn't feel like eating, a large glass of orange juice or a cup of tea will be enough—the appetite will return in due time. Don't force a tired athlete to eat a big meal heavy in protein. It's carbohydrates and minerals that are lacking, not protein.

The Pre-Practice Meal: If your athletic youngster rushes home from school and then out to practice, don't provide a big meal. A light, high-carbohydrate snack is better. The big meal can come afterwards, if desired.

The Nervous Athlete: Pre-game nerves often affect the stomach. Keep the meal light and easy to digest. (What was eaten the day before is the important thing, anyway.) Again, carbohydrates and citrus fruits are excellent.

The Box Lunch: Junk foods do provide some carbohydrate, but they don't do much for the balanced diet which the athlete requires. Make sure he or she takes a good, balanced lunch to school, with protein, carbohydrates and fruits, especially citrus, in the proportions mentioned earlier under general nutrition.

Vitamin Supplementation: This is a controversial point. But there is strong evidence that Vitamin C and B complex and iron supplementation will be useful for the athlete in endurance sports, particularly for girls. Most top coaches and athletes are strong believers in some form of vitamin supplementation, and a multipurpose vitamin pill probably will not be out of place.

Dr. L. Prokop of Austria reports that vitamin E has an effect on performance resulting from "an improvement of circulation and capillarization as well as through an improvement of oxygen utilization, of special significance for endurance performance". He adds that single vitamins often do not work well in isolation, and points to the "cooperation of different vitamins, each with the other, especially A, B_1, B_2, B_6, C and E."[2] Dr. Prokop seems to make a good case for multi-vitamin supplementation as part of the athlete's diet.

Heavy training is a stress situation, and scientific knowledge of the exact role of certain vitamins and minerals in combatting *specific* stresses is lacking. Further, individual athletes may have different requirements, depending on their sport, their strengths, and their weaknesses.

Gluttons Are Made, Not Born

Most parents are well aware of the role of nutrition in the growth and development of their child. Problems may arise when, by forcing children to eat foods they don't want but that we know are good for them, we establish habit patterns that may lead to obesity in later life.

Mother often starts the ball rolling by coaxing her baby to eat. She may equate a fat baby with a healthy baby – a bad mistake – or she may correlate food with love. Even very young children usually know when they've had enough, but they can be induced to eat more through coaxing and approval until they've emptied the plate. Or they may cry for a cuddle and some physical contact, and get a bottle of formula instead. Food then becomes part of a pattern of affection and solace.

How are we to develop proper eating habits? In their book, *Today's Child*, Dr. Elizabeth Chant Robertson and Dr. Margaret I. Wood, pediatricians at the Hospital for Sick Children in Toronto, suggest: "If he doesn't eat as much as you had hoped, don't try to coax, scold or wheedle him into eating more. He soon realizes that refusing some of his food disturbs you, and without a conscious thought on his part, he may find that spurning some of his food is more fun than eating it."[3]

As the child grows, junk foods are often used as rewards: candy for a good boy, to bed without supper for a bad one. He learns to use food, and usually the wrong kind of food, as a measure of his worth.

Parents should remember that the plump child often becomes the fat teenager and the obese adult. Take a look at your own relationship with your child and his diet. You may discover ways in which you, too, are encouraging him or her to look at food as a refuge or a source of love and esteem, rather than a source of nutrition to be enjoyed for its own sake.

DAILY FOOD GUIDE

Daily Requirements (unless otherwise specified)	Moderately Active Man	Moderately Active Woman	Child Age 4-6	Child Age 10-11	Girl Age 12-20	Boy Age 16-20
MILK (2-1/2 cups = 1 pint)	1½ cups	1½ cups	2½ cups	2½ cups	4 cups	4 cups
FRUITS Citrus, tomatoes and/or juice (one serving)	4.5 oz.	4.5 oz.	2.3 oz.	3.5 oz.	4.5 oz.	4.5 oz.
Other fruit (one serving)	4.5 oz.	4.5 oz.	2.3 oz.	3.5 oz.	4.5 oz.	4.5 oz.
VEGETABLES Potatoes (one serving)	6.8 oz.	6.8 oz.	3.4 oz.	6.8 oz.	6.8 oz.	9 oz.
Other–preferably yellow, green or raw (two servings)	4.5 oz. ea.	4.5 oz. ea.	2.3 oz. ea.	3.4 oz. ea.	4.5 oz. ea.	4.5 oz. ea.
BREAD (one slice equals one ounce)	9 oz.	4.5 oz.	4.5 oz.	7 oz.	8 oz.	12 oz.
BUTTEP OR FORTIFIED MARGARINE	1.7 oz.	1 oz.	.9 oz.	1.4 oz.	1.4 oz.	2.2 oz.
WHOLE GRAIN CEREAL (weekly amount)	8 oz.	8 oz.	4 oz.	8 oz.	8 oz.	10 oz.

153

MEAT AND ALTERNATIVES

Meat, poultry, fish (one serving per day)	36 oz. a wk.	28 oz. a wk.	10 oz. a wk.	16 oz. a wk.	20 oz. a wk.	36 oz. a wk.
Liver	3 oz. a wk.	4 oz. a wk.	2 oz. a wk.	3 oz. a wk.	3 oz. a wk.	3 oz. a wk.
Eggs (at least three times per week)	3 a wk.	6 a wk.	3 a wk.	3 a wk.	3 a wk.	3 a wk.
Cheese	6 oz. a wk.	3 oz. a wk.	1 oz. a wk.	3 oz. a wk.	4 oz. a wk.	4 oz. a wk.

VITAMIN D

400 International Units a day, for all growing persons, expectant and nursing mothers

EXTRAS AND OTHER FOODS (ounces per week)

Refined cereals (including noodles, polished rice, tapioca)	12	6	3	4	3	6
Fats	8	8	3	4	3	6
Sugar	10	10	2	4	4	10
Other Sweets	8	8	2	4	4	8
Tea, coffee, condiments as desired						

Source: *Reader's Digest*, November 1974. Adapted from Canada's Food Guide.

Note: People with weight problems, high blood pressure, etc., should consult a physician.

HOW TO CONTROL YOUR WEIGHT

More than 35 million North Americans are said to be suffering from obesity. On the average, most of them diet at least once a year, lose some weight, and are back to the starting point – or even fatter – a few months later.

There are two problems facing the person who had decided to lose weight: 1. losing weight, and 2. maintaining the desired weight (losing it permanently).

The first problem has been solved in a thousand different ways. There is probably more literature on diet than on almost any other subject dealing with the human condition. It ranges from down-to-earth, highly-researched documents by physiologists and physicians, to useful guides by nutritionists, to fad and crash diets involving everything from grapefruits to meditation.

The continued popularity of these diets indicates the need, and awareness of the need. It also hints at their central weakness: success, in many cases, is only temporary. (One bookseller in Los Angeles reported that, while diet books sold well, cookbooks outsold them 10 to 1.)

Some people can't seem to help being fat. Many psychologists now believe that persistent and uncontrollable overeating stems from unresolved emotional problems.

But with determination and common sense you can change habit patterns. As in fitness, there's no magic formula, no miracle diet which will enable you to shed pounds effortlessly. Let's look at some of the principles which have helped people who *have* lost weight, and *have* managed to stay slim.

1. Increase your physical activity so that calorie output equals or exceeds input.

2. Avoid crash or fad diets.

3. Reduce the load on your willpower as much as you can.

Increase your Physical Activity

You may not be eating too much – rather, you may not be getting enough exercise to burn up the calories you are taking in. Just 125 excess calories per day will produce a pound of fat a month (12 lbs. per year). Twenty minutes of fast walking per day would take care of that. This input-output ratio becomes increasingly important as you get older and your metabolism (which governs the rate at which you burn up calories) starts to slow down.

In addition to burning up calories, physical activity:

1. Boosts the basal metabolism. The rate at which you burn up calories not only rises during exercise, but stays higher for a long time afterwards (in some cases up to 48 hours if the exercise has been vigorous enough). Studies have also shown that severe cutbacks in calorie intake don't work as well as they should unless they are accompanied by increased physical activity because the metabolism reacts to starvation by slowing down. Consequently, weight loss starts to slow down as well.

2. Helps to regulate appetite. Many people believe that exercise increases appetite. It may, by heightening your feeling of well-being, enhance your enjoyment of food; however, inactivity more than activity is likely to make you feel hungry – you eat because you have no other outlet for the various drives which motivate you. This is sometimes called "displacement activity" – one activity substituted for another.

The basic problem of inactivity is that it does not *decrease* appetite. Calorie intake thus overwhelms output. A certain level of activity is required for the appetite control mechanism to function efficiently. Research has shown that strenuous exercise before a meal will actually decrease appetite.

Physical activity is good for you. Bad habits, it seems, are the only ones we enjoy. But think about this: If you exercise, you'll be able to enjoy your bad habits more.

Crash Diets

Crash diets which try to pare off 25 lbs. in a few weeks or fad diets which try out the latest gimmick in self-denial do not provide balanced nutrition in controlling weight, and they usually fail in the long run. Most people who go on crash diets have to start all over again a year later – just like the person who says he finds it easy to give up smoking because he's done it dozens of times.

"I don't have to worry about overeating. When I get too fat I eat nothing but grapefruit and alfalfa for a month, and I take it all off. I've done it before." Such people are usually just starting a diet, or just ending one. They are tired, irritable, and too fat. They become susceptible to infections and eventually their health suffers. That's one reason why most doctors do not approve of fad diets. Weight should not bounce up and down like a yoyo year after year.

Crash diets can become substitutes for a sensible life style in which balanced nutrition plays an important part. People who rely on crash diets never do lick their obesity problem. The average North American tries and abandons at least one diet a year. The crash diet syndrome is one of the causes: Why solve your weight problem by learning to eat right and exercise more when you can starve yourself thin tomorrow?

If, for medical reasons, you must lose a lot of weight in a short time, do it with your physician's supervision.

Willpower Made Easier

An effort of will is required to do something we don't want to do, particularly when it is contrary to established habits. Dieting – cutting down on one of life's chief pleasures – is particularly difficult. Why should we deprive ourselves of something we really enjoy?

It requires less willpower to do what we *have* to do. If the doctor were to tell us to take off 50 lbs. or die, most of us would diet. The strongest demand on the willpower makes itself felt as the target is approached.

When the sense of compulsion diminishes, it is easy to revert to old eating patterns. Then the real battle begins.

The inclination is to rationalize: "I've done it, now I can eat as I did before." This is one reason why crash diets fail: the person hasn't had time to establish *new habit patterns* – new attitudes and behaviors which are so ingrained that they become the natural way to think and behave. The dieter reverts to his old ways and is soon back in the same old blubber-laden boat.

Habits can be compared to athletic skill. When a tennis player corrects a fault – hitting backhands off the rear foot, for example – it takes a long time before the new technique becomes really ingrained. Under pressure, the old habit may reassert itself.

So, if we get into a stress situation, such as frustrations at the office, trouble at home or a row with a close friend, the pre-diet eating patterns come back. We may think it's temporary, but a real effort of will often is required to get back on the proper path.

"OK", you say. "I understand that. But how do I change my eating habits in the first place?"

The first step is to appreciate the need to lose weight, and make up your mind that it *has* to be done. The second is to realize that it's not just a matter of what you eat, but the way you eat. *Weight control is behavior control*. The third is to accept that new habits (skills) take time to establish. Setbacks should not to be more than a temporary discouragement, like a missed shot in tennis, but the long term objective—patterns of eating which meet your particular needs—should never be obscured.

Now we're ready to start looking at tricks and techniques that will help you.

The greatest single enemy of willpower in a diet is hunger – hunger so great it overwhelms you. The urge to eat becomes so strong that character and pride evaporate; you rationalize and find any number of reasons why dieting is not worthwhile and why it's all right to indulge yourself. After all, you're going to go back on a strict diet next week, or next month, or next year . . . Pretty soon you decide you're just a weakling; you simply *can't* diet.

All this is understandable. People who stay hungry day in and day out *are* overtaxing their willpower. There are several answers to help you beat the hunger syndrome.

1. *Make your objective realistic*. Unless you have been ordered to remove 50 lbs. immediately for medical reasons, don't try to do it all in a month. Remember that 12 lbs. lost over a year or six months, is just as much fat lost as 12 lbs. over a month, and it's a lot easier to achieve. First, figure out how much weight you've put on in the last year. Every pound represents about 3,500 calories. If you've put on 10 lbs., for example, you've taken in 35,000 calories more than you've been able to use up. That represents, on the average, 700 per week—only 100 per day!

Suppose you decide you only want to remove that extra 10 lbs., no more, no less. You have to eat just 100 calories less a day or increase your activity level by 100 calories. Easy enough. A good *brisk* walk for 20 minutes every day will take off the weight even without dieting!

Suppose your objective is 25 lbs. One year from now you're going to weigh 150 lbs. instead of 175, or 100 lbs. instead of 125. That's 250 calories per day. Fifteen minutes of jogging, 15 minutes of tennis, or half an hour of mowing the lawn with a hand mower, or an hour's walk, or any combination of these and similar activities will do it, again without dieting. The accompanying chart shows you the calorie burn-up of various common activities.

CALORIE BURN-UP OF VARIOUS ACTIVITIES

The figures shown here indicate the calories expended in an hour by a person ranging in weight from 125 lbs. (the lower figure) to 180 lbs. They are approximate since intensity of

ACTIVITY	CALORIE BURN-UP
Badminton or volleyball (moderate)	285–405
(vigorous)	488–695
Baseball (infield or outfield)	234–333
(pitching)	299–425
Basketball (moderate)	352–501
(vigorous)	495–703
Bowling (non-stop)	333–474
Cleaning windows	207–295
Conversation	92–130
Chopping weeds	367–521
Cycling (5.5 mph)	251–356
(13 mph)	537–764
Canoeing (4 mph)	352–500
Dancing (moderate)	209–297
(vigorous)	284–404
Gardening (including weeding)	295–416
Golf (twosome)	271–386
Handball	488–694
Hoeing, raking	235–334
Housework	203–289
Horseback riding (walking)	165–235
Making beds	196–278
Motorcycling	182–258
Mowing grass (power, self-propelled)	203–289
(power, pushed)	222–316
Pick and shovel work	335–475
Resting in bed	59–84
Rowing (pleasure)	251–356
(sculling machine, 20 strokes/min)	684–972
Running (5.5 mph)	536–764
(7 mph)	699–994
(9 mph, level)	777–1195
(up 4% grade)	959–1362
(12 mph)	984–1399
(in place, 140/min)	1222–1736
Sailing (light wind)	150–213
Sawing wood	391–556
Shovelling snow	389–556
Skating (moderate)	285–405
(vigorous)	513–729
Skiing (downhill)	483–687
(cross-country, 5 mph)	586–833
Sleeping	59–83
Standing (no activity)	71–100
(light activity)	122–173

ACTIVITY	CALORIE BURN-UP
Soccer	447–636
Squash	520–740
Swimming (crawl, 20 yds/min)	241–342
(50 yds/min)	532–757
Tennis (moderate)	347–492
(vigorous)	488–694
Table tennis	194–275
Television watching	60–72
Walking (2 mph)	176–249
(4-1/2 mph)	331–471
(up stairs)	869–1234
(down stairs)	333–474
Writing	92–130
Wrestling	634–914
Water skiing	391–556

movement will cause them to fluctuate up or down.

Unfortunately, it's not quite as clear sailing as it sounds. The principle would work if you didn't ever overindulge in high-calorie food and drink, and didn't miss a day's exercise. But one session of pizza with wine can put you a week behind schedule.

This is where the physical activity approach really becomes valuable. A vigorous fitness program 3 or 4 times a week, plus a walk every day, will not only help you get weight off fast, it will also increase your stamina and physical well-being and enable you to indulge yourself in food and drink on occasion without feeling guilty.

If you can decrease your calorie intake at the same time, you're well on the road to regaining the figure you had when you were in your 20s. Count calories for a couple of average weeks to see what you're consuming. Count everything – meals, snacks, drinks. No cheating. Keep a list. Good calorie-counting guides are available at most bookstores.

Now, how and what can you cut down? Sugar's a good place to start. It's high in calories and taken in excess is a health

hazard. Try your tea and coffee with an approved artificial sweetener or no sweetener at all. Cut down on canned foods. Eliminate desserts, mayonnaise (except the calorie-reduced kind), chocolate bars, nuts, and soft drinks (except the low-cal type).

Trim the fat off meat. A gram of fat contains twice as many calories as a gram of protein, and you'll be eliminating a source of saturated fatty acids (containing cholesterol) as well. Reduce the size of the portions you eat. With very little effort you can probably eliminate 300 or 400 calories.

You have the choice of trying for quick weight reduction by dieting and exercising every day, or you can make it a longer project by either exercising or dieting every day. You can set a 2-month objective, or you can set a 6-month objective.

Whichever method you choose, make the change permanent, a new life style. Do not regard it as a temporary measure to be abandoned when you've achieved your objective. What you want are new living skills which keep you physically fit and trim.

It's probably best to make your objective a long-term one. Set your target for a year ahead. Decide how much exercise you can enjoyably handle – remember that you'll need at least 3 exercise sessions per week for a significant fitness benefit, and set yourself a calorie objective that's within range of your willpower.

2. *Change your snack pattern:* Snacks, mid-morning coffee breaks, and restaurant meals can sabotage even the best diet intentions. Develop an "anti-fat brigade" – foods and beverages which are relatively low in calories and high in nutrition. A couple of biscuits with a 3 x 3-inch slice of cheddar would be only 150 calories (without butter or you can use low-cal margarine). That's the same number of calories as 15 potato chips, but much more satisfying and nutritious. Drink coffee or tea black or use an approved artificial sweetener. Carry some with you. A soft drink should be of the low-cal type.

THE ANTI-FAT BRIGADE

These are some foods and snacks which can satisfy a craving for food without providing too many calories. They are useful for those occasions when your diet seems to be collapsing around you, when your yearning for food is stronger than your willpower.

Most snacks these days are high-sugar foods which can upset the sugar balance of the body – they actually increase the desire for food so that you overeat at the next meal. (The reasons for this are discussed in

Chapter 9, *Fitness at Work Too*, in the section on coffee breaks.) Protein snacks provide more "energy fuel" in the long run, and do not have the same effect on your hunger mechanism.

A dill pickle, by the way, can sharpen up a snack, provide a little something extra to eat – and it's only 15 calories!

Eat your snack slowly. It'll last longer, and seem like more. And even in the anti-fat brigade, moderation is the watchword. One piece of cheese has only 100 calories, 4 pieces 400.

Vegetables	CALORIES
Lettuce (large serving)	25
Celery (1 cup)	40
Cabbage (1/2 cup cooked)	40
(1/2 cup fresh, shredded)	13
Turnip (1/2 cup)	20
Carrots (1/2 cup cooked)	30
(1/2 cup raw, shredded)	25
Cauliflower (1/2 cup)	40
Green or yellow beans (1/2 cup)	30
Onions (1 medium)	30
Tomatoes (1 medium)	30
Water cress (1 bunch)	20
Radishes (10 medium)	30
Green peas (1/2 cup drained)	45
Parsnips (1/2 cup)	45
Olives (2 large)	25
Dill pickle (medium)	15
Kale (1/2 cup steamed)	30
Asparagus (1/2 cup)	25
Bean sprouts (1 cup)	32
Beet greens (1/2 cup)	33
Broccoli (1/2 cup)	20
Brussels sprouts (1/2 cup)	20
Squash (1/2 cup)	18
Cucumbers (14 thin slices)	14

Fruit (fresh)	CALORIES
Apple (medium)	70–80
Orange (medium)	60–70
Grapefruit (1/2 medium)	100
Apricots (1 medium, fresh)	80
(5 halves dried)	50
Raspberries (1/2 cup)	45
Strawberries (1/2 cup)	40
Blueberries (1/2 cup)	40
Loganberries (1/2 cup)	50
Peaches (1 medium)	50
Pears (1 medium)	50
Pineapples (1-3/4" slice)	30
Plums (1 medium)	15
Cantaloupe (1/2 medium)	30
Bananas (1 medium)	100

Bread	
White	50-60
Rye	60-70
Whole wheat (60%)	55
(100%)	75
Melba toast	20
Crackers (1 soda or saltine)	25

Soups (large bowl)

	CALORIES
Consomme	25
Bouillon	25
Clear tomato	80–100
Chicken with noodles (strained)	60–70
Clam bouillon	25–30

Snacks

Cottage cheese (5 tbsp. skim milk)	100
Cheese, cheddar (3x3x1/4")	100
Crab meat (1/2 cup)	65
Lobster meat (1/2 cup)	75
Shrimp (2/3 cup, canned)	40
Sauerkraut (1/2 cup)	20
Skim milk (1 glass)	80–90
Puffed rice (1 cup)	45

Candy

Jujubes (8 small)	32

Calorie-reduced foods, beverages, and condiments

As advertised on container

Other foods and snacks

Check your calorie counter for additions to this list

3. *Watch out for "danger" foods:* Certain foods and beverages can throw your program haywire. Watch out for them. Chocolates, nuts, cookies, malted milk, soft drinks, mayonnaise, salami, high-sugar and fat foods add up very quickly. The more of them you can cut out of your diet, the more you'll be able to eat other low-calorie foods. Look at the accompanying list of danger foods and check a calorie counter for others; keep track of how often you eat them. See how many you can reduce in portion or size, or eliminate completely.

Of course, if you get your calorie count well under control through lots of exercise and balanced nutrition, you don't have to worry as much if you indulge yourself occasionally – a bonus for the balanced diet.

DANGER LIST

Chocolate (1 small bar)	250
Cashew nuts (4)	100
Cookie (1)	100
Ice cream (1/2 cup)	260
Chocolate malted milk (large glass)	460
Mayonnaise (1 tablespoon)	100
Salami (1 average slice)	132
Waffle (1)	250
Peanuts (1/4 cup – 2 ounces)	200
Peanut butter (4 tablespoons)	375
Macaroni and cheese (1 cup)	470

Consult your calorie counter for additions to this list.

4. *Smaller meals, but more of them:* According to Dr. Jean Mayer, one of the world's most respected nutritionists, a safe and effective method of controlling weight is eating smaller portions on a schedule which averts the development of excessive hunger:

5 small meals a day rather than 1 or 2 big ones.

Many people, for example, do without breakfast. By mid-morning, hunger pangs and low blood-sugar levels drive them to eat a high-carbohydrate snack. They're still hungry by lunchtime and may overeat. In North America, supper is by custom the large meal of the day, so there's psychological pressure to eat too much again.

A medium-sized breakfast, a protein snack, a small but nutritious lunch, and another protein snack will probably set you up for a sensible supper and enable you to keep your calorie count low enough so that you can have another snack in the evening.

5. *Eat slowly:* The process of satiety—the body's reaction that you've had enough—takes a little time. If you eat fast, by the time you feel full you've actually eaten too much: haste makes waist.

6. *Don't eliminate carbohydrates:* Too few carbohydrates in the diet will create fatigue and make you irritable. Any diet with an imbalance of essential nutrients should be avoided. Dr. Jean Mayer recommends that the diet of the average, relatively inactive person should contain: protein, 20 per cent; fat, 30 per cent (saturated animal fat only 5 per cent); carbohydrate, 50 per cent (refined sugars only 5 per cent).[4]

Cut down the refined sugars, and get your carbohydrates from natural sources like fresh fruits and vegetables. Most canned goods contain refined sugar which is used as a preservative.

7. *Moderate amounts of salt:* Except for those with certain medical conditions, a salt-free diet is neither recommended nor necessary. Use salt in moderation, and avoid foods and snacks which are highly salted in their preparation. Decreasing salt intake can help boost your morale, since the body will retain less water and you will *appear* to have lost weight. Do not reduce salt levels too far, however, if you exercise vigorously during hot weather. The salts and trace elements which you lose in your sweat must be replaced.

How frequently should you check your weight? When you are on a diet, the bathroom scale is an invaluable guide to progress; but the scale will not tell you the truth if you haunt it every day. Weigh yourself in the nude once a week before breakfast. Body weight fluctuates from morning to night and from day to day since weight loss is uneven. There may be no change at all for a few days, then a sudden drop. You may even gain a pound or two. Do not be discouraged. If you are sticking to your diet and exercising, you are losing weight and the scales will eventually register the happy fact.

Diet Aids

Diet aids such as low-calorie foods and beverages can be extremely useful if they are not abused. But these and certain other items, such as bulk-producing agents and hormone injections, should be approached with care.

Calorie-reduced foods and beverages; Because these foods are described as "low" in calories, many people fool themselves about quantity. They pile on low-cal mayonnaise, or drink 5 low-cal soft drinks, or help themselves to a few handfuls of low-cal mints, and are soon getting just as many calories as before.

Soft drink manufacturers are planning to continue with low-cal beverages despite the ban on saccharin, using alternative sweeteners. Even before the ban, however, one well-known diet drink contained 3.5 calories per fluid ounce. Six tins a day would add up to 210 calories, so obviously some self-control has to be exercised, especially if calorie counts go up in the saccharin-substitute drinks.

The same holds true for such "diet" foods as remain on the market after the ban. Many of these foods are desserts, candies, jams, and cookies which are no substitute for balanced nutrition and can be misleading if you don't read the label carefully. An 8 oz. can of low-calorie fruit cocktail, for example, could contain up to 100 calories; fresh fruit, which is cheaper, would have about the same number and be better for you.

A 4 oz. serving of low-calorie pudding might have 59 calories if made with skim milk, and 94 if whole milk is used.

Beware of so-called dietetic foods as a reducing aid. The sugar has been reduced or removed to make them acceptable to diabetics. But in many cases it has been replaced with fat which contains twice as many calories per ounce as does sugar. Some dietetic foods, therefore, have far more calories than you may think they have. Read the label. If it doesn't provide a calorie count, avoid the product.

With these reservations, reduced-calorie foods and beverages can be a tremendous help in bulking up your diet and giving you a feeling of satiety without adding too many calories. Some willpower is required to avoid overdoing the quantities and to get used to the flavors.

Artificial sweeteners: Studies have shown that saccharin ingested in high quantities can cause cancer in rats. While there is no direct evidence that it causes cancer in humans, its controlled use will require dieters to look for alternate, approved sweeteners. Remember, however, that while there is doubt about the government's findings regarding saccharin, there is *no* question that sugar used in the quantities to which many people are accustomed is a definite health hazard.

Appetite suppressants: These result in only small additional weight losses, according to the Food and Drug Administration in the United States. Those which are amphetamines can be habit forming. Avoid them. Nor are hormone injections considered

to be effective in the treatment of obesity.

Before-meal candies are advertised as appetite depressants and are supposed to increase blood sugar levels so that the dieter can push aside tempting desserts. They contain vitamin and mineral supplements as well. But *Consumer Reports* pointed out that in the recommended dose of one or two candies, there is unlikely to be an appreciable rise in blood sugar, and there is no guarantee that it will depress appetite. Two candies equal 50 calories – not much of an exchange if it doesn't work.

Bulk-producing agents containing methyl cellulose which swells when it comes in contact with water are supposed to reduce hunger contractions. Again, this does not guarantee a reduction in appetite. Appetite is based on other things besides hunger, including learned patterns, sensations of well-being and enjoyment, reactions to situations (it's one o'clock, time to eat), and the appearance and smell of food.

Dr. Jean Mayer suggests that raw carrots, apples, celery, and raw salads are superior bulk-producing agents and are more palatable and nutritious then methyl cellulose products. They also slow down the meal and provide *time* for satiety – the body's "I've had enough" reaction – which artificial bulk producers fail to do.

Formula diets: So-called formula diets such as Metrecal and others provide adequate nutritional value with a low calorie count. In fact, they are *so* low in calories it's unwise to tackle them without the advice of your physician, and research has shown that more people fail on this form of diet than succeed. It's monotonous, expensive, and does not really provide a satiety value. When supplemented with other foods, it tends to lose its value.

In the long run, good nutrition with adequate exercise is the only formula that really works. Diet aids, used intelligently, can help to provide certain shortcuts, but they are not substitutes for sensible nutrition.

Gaining Weight

In the hubub about obesity, the individual who wants to gain weight is frequently forgotten, yet underweight is a definite problem. Thin people may appear bony and pale, and lack strength for demanding physical tasks. In reality, they are probably fitter and healthier than those who are obese. But pride and social pressure dictate that they fill out their clothes, especially bathing suits, better than they do.

Athletes often wish to add bulk in the form of muscle. Strength is a common denominator of sports efficiency, and while most events, with the exception of weight throws and lifting, do not demand a great deal of bulk, strength gains often are accompanied by muscle hypertrophy (increase in size). Slender people usually have a genetic endowment – a body type – which predisposes them to lack of muscle bulk. They can never get into the super heavyweight class, and chances are they'll never add enough fat to play Santa Claus without a pillow. However, they can become extremely strong and they can, through determined eating, gain a considerable amount of weight.

Most thin people do not risk the health hazards that face the obese, provided their thinness is not due to a medical problem, and provided they do not drop below certain limits. However, if they do want to gain weight, they need more muscle, not more fat. That's why simply eating your way into a higher weight category is usually a mistake.

First, if you are excessively thin, check with your physician to make sure there's nothing medically wrong.

Second, check your diet. It may be that you do not eat enough to keep ahead of your metabolism. Don't try to bulk up with junk foods containing "dead" calories (calories without nutritional value such as those found in sugar). Concentrate on such nutritious items as nuts, dried fruit, milk and cheese, lima and soya beans, vegetable oils.

If you dislike big, heavy meals, accompany each meal with liquids which are high in both calories and nutrition; drink them between meals as well. High-calorie "liquid meals" which will give you 1,200 or more calories per day without overtaxing your stomach capacity are now available. By the way, while a weight-gaining program should be rich in protein, there's no evidence that *extremely* large quantities of protein can be utilized by the body.

Third, get started on a program of physical activity which will develop muscle bulk. (Weight training or some form of isometric exercise is the quickest way to do this.)

Fourth, do not go on a high-calorie diet without exercising. If the increase in weight is fat rather than muscle, you will be subject to all the health hazards of obesity.

If you are a woman, remember that attractive curves are produced not by fat but by muscle. Fat by itself merely congregates in all the wrong places. You don't have to look like a shotputter, but you do need enough muscle to fill out the hollows and give you a rounded appearance.

Don't overdo calorie-burning activities such as jogging, tennis, or all-night dancing. Slow down a bit and get extra rest and sleep. Chances are you're a fairly tense individual anyway, so learn to relax and take it a bit easier. Try some of the relaxation drills in Chapter 8. They'll ease tension and help you lead a more casual life style.

When you reach the proportions you are seeking, ease off on high-calorie foods and modify your exercise habits. But don't abandon the whole program. Muscles disappear almost as fast as they're created, and before you know it, the mirror will start showing you that same linear physique you started with.

8

How To Reduce Tension and Learn to Relax

Relaxation is a skill. Like hitting a tennis ball or skiing down a hill, it is a coordination of mind and muscles. And, like any physical skill, it can be learned by anyone who wants to do so and is willing to spend the time and effort.

Why is it important to learn to relax?

The reasons are many, with far-reaching implications for your body and your emotions. Relaxation tends to reduce blood pressure and the workload on the heart. It conserves energy, since tense muscles are working muscles, and it helps to settle down the nervous system so that your anxieties are less intense, you are slower to anger and not as likely to be upset by little things.

Your ability to handle stress is improved. Emotion is less likely to cloud your judgment, enabling you to assess important situations realistically. Daily tasks become less fatiguing. Your reserve of physical and emotional energy is thus increased and with it enjoyment of your social life. You have a greater reserve to handle emergencies.

Most important of all, inability to relax creates tension, a mortal enemy of physical and emotional fitness and health.

Tension, an involuntary tightening of the muscles, is usually a byproduct of stress and anxiety. Sometimes it is caused by our emotions, sometimes by an improperly coordinated effort to perform a physical activity. It is part of the body's attempt to prepare itself to withstand a threat of some kind—what Dr. Hans Selye calls a stressor. The so-called threat may be highly visible, such as an important business meeting or an impending deadline; or it may be obscure and have as its expression feelings of anxiety, either residual and ongoing, or worry about some specific event in the distant future.

STRESS, ANXIETY, AND TENSION

Stress, anxiety and tension—many people use the words interchangeably. In reality, they are labels for three states which are related, yet different. Stress can produce both anxiety and tension; anxiety and tension create stress.

What's the difference, then? Stress is a temporarily induced physiological and psychological imbalance caused by an event which the individual regards as a possible danger. It is the state which exists between the time the stressor exerts its influence and the body begins to adapt to it.

Anxiety is an emotional state; it can even be a personality characteristic of the chronic worrier who expects things to go wrong. He or she has a general sense of fear and foreboding, a sense of failure, lack of confidence, and uncertainty.

Tension is the average individual's physical reaction to stress and anxiety.

One solution is to teach the muscles a relaxation reflex so that when the stress occurs the body's adaptive response is an easing of tension rather than an increase — like the champion athlete who seizes a split second opportunity and scores the winning goal, rather than the loser who freezes or "chokes" and loses his chance.

A relaxation reflex can also help to release the tension which is created by anxiety, and the coordination tension which results from misdirected physical effort. The stiff, aching muscles a typist may get in the neck and shoulders is one example of the latter. The shoulder muscles should not be directly involved in the typing, but the mind tells them to tighten up anyway.

Stress

Dr. Hans Selye is the pioneer of work in this field and has broadened our understanding of the nature of stress. Selye has formulated as the basis of his theories a "general adaptation syndrome". This is how it works.

Heat, cold, fear, and countless other factors create a form of stress which requires the body to adapt to their influences. This adaptation consists of three stages: 1. alarm, 2. resistance and adaptation, 3. exhaustion.

The alarm stage occurs when your body realizes that a stressor is present. Suppose it is heat. You feel hot, and the body adapts by perspiring. The exhaustion state occurs when the body, unable to overcome the heat stress, suffers dehydration and heat stroke.

It is at this third stage that physiological malfunctions (breakdowns, illnesses) are likely to occur. According to Selye: "Some diseases in which stress plays a particularly important role are high blood pressure, cardiac accidents, gastric or duodenal ulcers . . . and various types of mental disturbances."[1]

The body's reaction to stress is often called the "fight or flight" response because the physical changes which take place prepare it to fight the stress, or to retreat from it. Adrenalin and other chemicals and hormones are released, heart rate increases, the senses are sharpened and concentrated, and the muscles receive a quick charge of energy. In severe stress, the pupils of the eye dilate, the mouth goes dry, perspiration begins, and gastric processes stop.

These reactions, in varying degrees, go on all day. The stressor may be at a low level, as for example a knock on the door, or the ring of the telephone. It may increase suddenly in intensity when the caller is your boss, for example.

Some people are able to release muscular tension quickly when the stress passes, but most remain tense to a greater or lesser degree. Their muscles are unable to relax completely after the stress subsides, and the tension tends to accumulate. This residual tension can be a serious problem. It becomes in itself a severe form of stress which, unless it is released, may bring the individual to the exhaustion stage. The manifestations vary from person to person. Some of us get ulcers, others develop nervous tics, or have heart attacks and breakdowns. Early symptoms include irritability, sudden bursts of temper, depression, and insomnia. This is why relaxation is a skill we should all try to acquire. The muscles can be taught to relax; once they learn how, it becomes as much a reflex action as was the tension response.

How does stress cause such problems as heart trouble?

The late Dr. Wilhelm Raab of the University of Vermont was one of the foremost researchers investigating this area of human fallibility. He developed the V-S Ratio theory which illustrates how stresses can damage the heart muscle.

V-S refers to the two basic forms of stimulation which the heart receives. V stands for the vagus nerve through which the parasympathetic nervous system sends its messages to the heart. This is the one which is activated by physical activity and, according to Dr. Raab, its influences are beneficial. S stands for the sympathetic nervous system. Factors such as anger, fear, grief, tension, smoking, worry, and alcohol stimulate the heart via this route and cause the release of chemical by-products which have a detrimental effect, particularly on the heart.

Further, Dr. Raab believes that only vagus stimulation of the heart can counteract the stress created by sympathetic stimulation. There should be a balance between V and S for the heart muscle to remain healthy.

The active athlete probably will get about 80 per cent of his heart stimulation from V factors, and only 20 per cent from the S side. The highly-pressured business executive, however, is on the other end of the teeter-totter. Physical activity provides only 20 per cent (or less) of his heart stimulation; the rest of it comes from worry, anxiety, tension, and other stress factors. Most of us are somewhere in between. Judging from the incidence of coronary heart disease, however, many of us are edging toward the wrong side of the scale.

The less regular physical activity we get, the higher the degree of stress will be on the heart, particularly from factors such as anxiety and tension.

Individuals vary in their ability to tolerate stress. Selye refers to this quality as "adaptation energy". People who have a lot of it can withstand a great deal more stress than those who do not. On the other hand, even the high-tolerance individual can run into trouble if he or she allows the stress level to exceed the tolerance level. Adaptation energy is not limitless; it becomes depleted, particularly as we grow older.

A comfortable degree of stress is essential. It spurs creativity and productivity; it makes life worth living because it requires us to strive and achieve. Says Selye: "Few things are as frustrating as complete inactivity, the absence of any stimulus, any challenge to which you could react."[2]

All of us run into periods in which we are in danger of being overwhelmed by our stresses – sudden unexpected responsibilities, a death in the family, a personal crisis. We may experience headaches, insomnia, gastric upsets, and excessive fatigue. We may become easily irritated and develop skin disorders.

Rest and recreation help. (Selye calls it "the healing stress of diversion".) But if the high-stress situation continues for long periods, it leads to "adaptation failure". Then even an insignificant factor can be overwhelming and leave you seriously ill.

Regular physical activity provides one line of defence. "There is a nonspecific resistance (to stressors) that can be acquired by making continuous but moderate demands upon our organs, for example, our muscles and brain," Selye writes in *Stress Without Distress* (p. 74).

The second and equally important safeguard is to learn the art of physical relaxation, the ability to release the tension in the muscles which is one of the symptoms of stress. The symptom is not the disease, but relieving this particular symptom will go a long way toward fighting off the effects of the disease and will also help to maintain the body's adaptive energy.

Anxiety and tension, then, are major partners in the stress syndrome. In order to know how to combat stress, it is a good idea to understand exactly what they are and how they affect your health.

Anxiety

Anxiety is an emotional state which often is an integral part of your personality. It stimulates the sympathetic nervous system, it may overwork the endocrine glands, and it keeps the body in a *constant* state of readiness to meet a threat. This is why highly-anxious persons are usually extremely tense.

This is dispositional anxiety; it is a part of your makeup. There is also an anxiety response to specific situations: an exam, a business meeting, any event which you anticipate will be difficult to handle. Once the situation passes, this anxiety diminishes but dispositional anxiety remains.

One common form of anxiety which is extremely inimical to health and zest for living is "failure anxiety" (also referred to as an inferiority complex). By visualizing failure and its consequences, we become overconcerned with the *results* of our actions instead of the performance. The athlete's fear of failure causes him "to choke", to tense up and become disoriented, and he fails. For example, the pro golfer on the 18th green is lining up the winning putt and instead of concentrating on the lie of the green and the mechanics of what he's doing, he thinks: "What if I miss? I'll lose all that money." More often than not, he misses. Psychologists term this a self-fulfilling prophecy: the golfer has predicted his own failure.

Coaches recognize this situation and have various ways of combatting it. They may tell their athletes: "Think of what you're going to do, rather than how well you're going to do." or "Concentrate on keeping your head down." Sports psychologists are now used in many countries to help athletes with positive mental images so that the possibility of failure does not enter their minds. The anxiety and fear are still there, but the buildup to the big event follows a carefully organized mental pattern which, for that particular athlete, keeps the anxiety from interfering with his neuromuscular and psychological behavior.

Tension

A certain degree of anxiety is essential for sheer survival. Driving in heavy traffic would be dangerous, for example, if the driver were completely unconcerned and complacent. But if he dwelt too much on the possibility of failure – in this case, of having an accident – he would become mentally and physically rigid. His thinking would be less clear and organized; he would develop muscular tension and become, in effect, prone to the accident he feared.

Tension is not just a vague feeling of tightness accompanied by headaches or dizziness, although these symptoms often result from tension. It is a general involuntary tightening of the muscles throughout the body in response to a stressor – the preparation to meet the enemy. In the early days of mankind, this reaction was vital. It was the fight or flight response which kept man alive. We do not have the same opportunities to respond physically that our ancestors had. Even the problems are different; usually they are more mental than physical. The reaction, however, remains the same – muscle tension.

Tension is the greatest single restrictor of physical efficiency. Because it is non-specific and occurs throughout the body, it drains us of energy, damages our circulatory system, and interferes with the coordinated action of our neuromuscular system.

There are two basic types of tension: coordination tension and affective tension. Coordination tension is usually related to the performance of skills which have not yet been completely learned and is gradually eliminated as skills improve through practice and experience. It does not disappear completely, however; even in trained athletes it can restrict movement and spoil efficiency. Tension interferes with coordination by diverting the flow of messages from the brain to the muscles and back again. Muscles which ought not to be tense grow tense and the biofeedback mechanisms become confused. You can thread a needle, sink a putt, or play a violin much better when you are relaxed than when you are tense.

The second type, known as affective tension, is created by habits, attitudes, and thought patterns. More difficult to eradicate and also more injurious to health, it is linked to such psychosomatic ailments as ulcers, headaches, and heart-circulatory diseases. This is the form of tension we will be discussing.

Affective tension is insidious. It sneaks up on you. In the early stages, you usually are not aware of its presence. You may be sitting in your car, fighting rush hour traffic and gripping the wheel so hard your knuckles are white. Your shoulders are hunched up around your ears and your stomach muscles are knotted – but you don't even notice it.

The harder you press to accomplish something, the more your affective tension may tie you up. You could be typing fast to finish a letter before quitting time, or trying excessively hard to convince a prospective buyer. In your concentration on what you are doing, you don't even notice how much your muscles are contracting, but your body is actually under a heavy workload. No wonder you often feel worn out at the end of a day of hard mental and emotional effort. Tense, contracted muscles are working muscles which are burning up energy and vitality.

Unfortunately, tense muscles have yet another effect. By exerting pressure on nearby blood vessels, they interfere with circulation. The restricted flow of oxygen to the brain and to the body's cells, causes dizziness as well as vague aches and pains of fatigue. Blood pressure becomes elevated as well.

Most people develop affective tension in the neck and shoulders; however, it may also occur in the jaw, the hands, or the stomach. Everybody seems to have a particular tension target area.

Unless it is released, tension tends to persist and accumulate. The buildup of tension becomes a severe stress and major problems begin – ulcers, hypertension, or heart-circulatory disorders.

Fortunately, there are solutions. If there were not, all compulsive achievers – businessmen, artists, industrialists, politicians, stockbrokers, scientists and the rest – would drop like flies after a year or two (instead of waiting until they reach their 40s).

Willpower alone is not the answer. You cannot force a muscle to relax. In fact, the harder you try the more tension you are likely to create, unless you have certain skills at your command.

TENSION RELEASE – THE TECHNIQUE

There are six major steps to relaxation:

1. *Knowledge:* learning what tension is.

2. *Recognition:* learning the difference between the feeling of tension and the feeling of relaxation.

3. *Control:* learning the fundamental skill of relaxing the various muscle groups.

4. *Program:* organizing a relaxation program suitable for your particular problems, available time, and inclinations.

5. *Daily Practice:* applying to your daily activities the skill of relaxing which you have developed. This will include learning special tricks and techniques for particular tension crises in your life: speeches, arguments, important sales contacts, big sports events.

6. *Teaching:* teaching what you know to at least one other person. This may not seem important, but instructing someone else – a member of your family, a friend or a business associate – will not only help them but will develop your own skill and understanding.

Steps 1 and 2—Getting Started

Since we've already discussed the meaning of tension, we can begin at step 2: learning to recognize the difference in the way the muscles feel when they are tense and when they are relaxed. To achieve this, you must consciously induce tension in yourself so that you can recognize the *feeling* of tension in the muscle.

To learn the skill of staying loose under pressure you must practise, as you would have to practise a difficult dive or a gymnastic routine. This will take time and dedication, of course. Eventually, the body will begin to develop a conditioned reflex, so that whenever tension begins to accumulate, its automatic response will be relaxation.

RECOGNITION DRILL

This can be done while standing, sitting, or even lying down. Take a moderately deep breath and tense up all the muscles throughout your body. Feel the tension; examine it. Hold for 3 to 5 seconds, relax, and exhale with a long, easy sigh. As you exhale, let all the muscles go as loose and relaxed as possible. Feel the tension seeping out of the muscles. Repeat 6 to 8 times.

It helps the biofeedback mechanisms if you create mental images: "This is tension, this is what tension feels like." As you relax, say to yourself: "This is relaxation, this is how it feels to be loose, this is what I want." Examine yourself to see if there are any areas which haven't relaxed completely; let them go loose too, and then even looser. Conjure up a mental image of complete relaxation.

So far you have been tensing and relaxing the body generally. Now concentrate on specific parts: the neck, shoulders, hands, arms, legs, stomach. Isolate each one and do the recognition drill. Pay special attention to those muscles which appear to be your particular tension targets.

To finish the drill, lie or sit "loose and easy". Let everything go, exhaling with a long sigh, allowing all your muscles to collapse. Picture everything inside your body turning to jelly. Relaxing is not a forced movement—it is "giving up". You stop trying and collapse.

This, then, is your preliminary control drill. It may be done whenever you feel tense, and at intervals during the day when you have a moment or two to yourself. You may relax the whole body, or select a muscle group or two and work on that. The oftener you do it, the better.

Continue this recognition drill for about two weeks, or until you are honestly convinced that you can control your muscles, and that you are becoming conscious of tension when it starts to creep up on you.

During this initial period of recognition and control, make an effort to become aware of tension not only in yourself but in other

people too. Look for tense individuals, and those who are relaxed. Notice the differences in their behavior and the way in which they move and react.

Step 3 – Control

At the end of two weeks, if you've done your drills regularly and properly, you will have started to associate the process of conscious relaxation with your general activities.

You should now replace the basic recognition and control drill with the following more advanced control drill which is designed to increase your skill in relaxing particular parts of the body and to establish a finer, deeper muscle control. It should be done in its entirety at least once a day, preferably at bedtime. If you can find the time, a session, or a partial session, first thing in the morning will help you start the day feeling relaxed.

The drill is done in three sections: rotation, collapsing, and breathing.

A. ROTATION DRILLS

Tension is both the cause and the result of inflexibility in the joints. If you are to feel freedom and ease of movement, you must be fairly loose in all the important "hinges" which permit movement. The spine, upon which the entire body is suspended, is a particularly important area. So is the midsection, where excess tension can contribute to several functional disorders as well as vague aches, pains, and discomfort.

These drills can be done in sequence to form a special program aimed at limbering the joints, or individually as part of a basic relaxation program.

 FOOT AND LOWER LEG ROTATION

Lie on back or sit in an easy chair and rotate your feet slowly and easily in large circles, 7 or 8 times in each direction. Breathe deeply from the stomach, trying to achieve additional relaxation with each exhale. Now lift your knees and rotate the lower legs in large circles, nice and loose with the feet hanging limply. Do 7 or 8 each way.

 ELBOWS UP TORSO TWIST

Stand with feet comfortably apart, knees slightly bent and elbows out to your sides at shoulder height, forearms hanging loosely. Twist your torso around to the right as far as possible, turning your head so that you finish up looking behind you. Now twist around to the opposite side, letting the arms follow your torso around, swinging loosely with the hands and wrists relaxed. Move at a comfortable pace, getting a maximum amount of turn but not forcing yourself or creating excess muscular effort. Do 10 turns to each side.

 LATERAL HIP SWING

Swing your hips from one side to the other, moving slowly and letting your muscles go loose and limp. Continue for about half a minute.

 ELBOW ROTATION

Standing with feet comfortably apart, bend your arms at right angles and raise the elbows out to the sides to shoulder height. Your forearms should be parallel to the ground with hands hanging loosely. Move the elbows back as far as you can, and rotate them high and forward, making a large circle. Repeat 7 or 8 times in each direction.

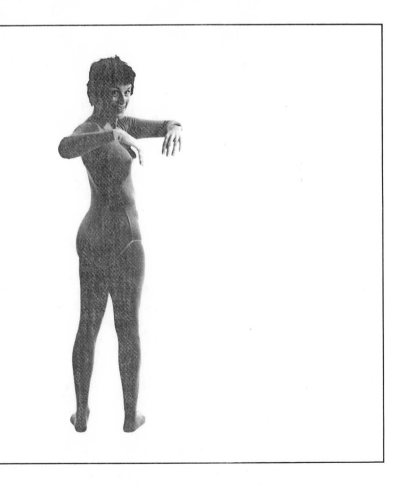

Elbows Up Torso Twist

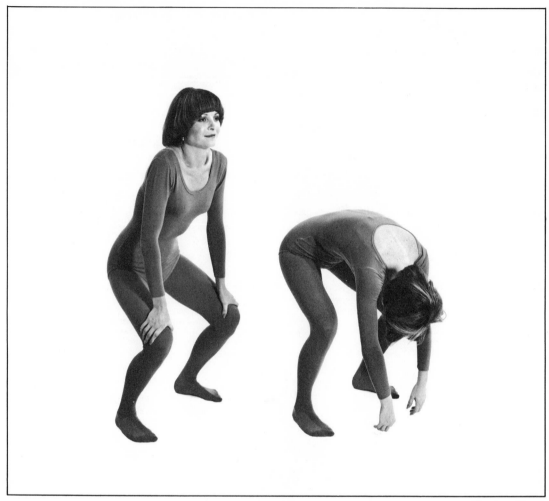

Monkey Slump

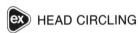 **HEAD CIRCLING**

In a sitting position, let your chin drop to your chest. Keeping the neck relaxed, rotate your head in big circles, first one way and then the other. Your jaw should hang open loosely. You may hear some creaking and popping noises. Don't be alarmed. This simply indicates that the area needs a bit of loosening up. Do 6 or 7 easy circles in each direction.

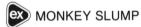 **MONKEY SLUMP**

Stand with feet comfortably apart and knees slightly bent. Place hands on knees, breathe in deeply, and moderately tense up the muscles throughout the body. Now exhale with a long, slow sigh, letting your hands slip from your knees and your body slump forward until the hands touch the floor and the chest rests on the thighs.

Stay in this slump for 3 to 5 seconds, then slowly return to the starting position and repeat 6 times.

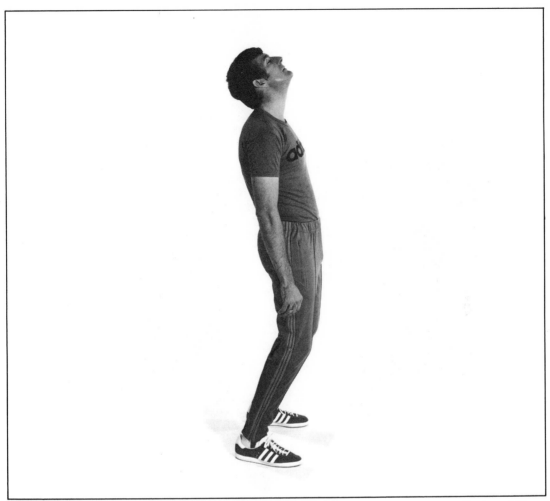

Backward Slump

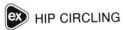 HIP CIRCLING

Stand with feet comfortably apart. Keeping your knees straight, move your hip and groin area in big circles by swinging the hips forward, to the side, and back. Move slowly and easily 5 or 6 times to the right. Reverse.

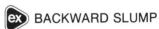 BACKWARD SLUMP

Stand comfortably. Let your head and upper body slump slowly backwards as far as you can without falling over. The knees should bend and the head flop back loosely. Repeat 5 or 6 times.

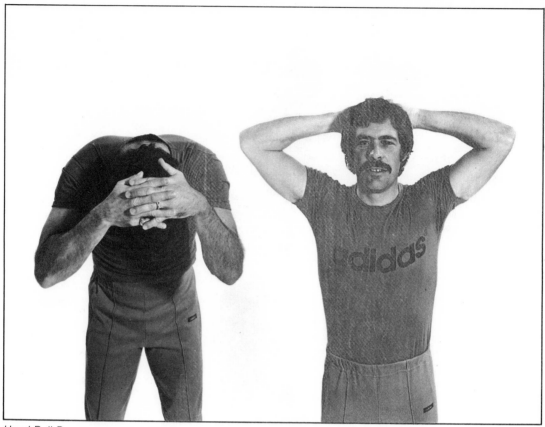

Head Pull Down

 HEAD PULL DOWN

With hands clasped high on back of skull, let head drop forward toward chest. *Slowly* exert pressure on the head so that neck and upper body round forward into chest. Return slowly to starting position and repeat 5 or 6 times.

 FOREARM ROTATION

Lie on back with arms bent, forearms pointing up in the air. Rotate your forearms in large circles, first one way and then the other, keeping them loose and floppy.

 LEG ROTATION

Lie on your back. Lift your left leg 6 to 8 inches, keeping the knee stiff, and cross it over the right leg as far as it will go. Then bend the left knee and bring it up toward your right shoulder, keeping the right leg flat and straight. Cross back to the left until the knee touches the floor. Straighten it out and return to the starting position. Do 3 or 4 circles with each leg to loosen up the hip and pelvic area.

 JAW ROTATION

Let the lower jaw hang loosely and rotate it 6 times in each direction.

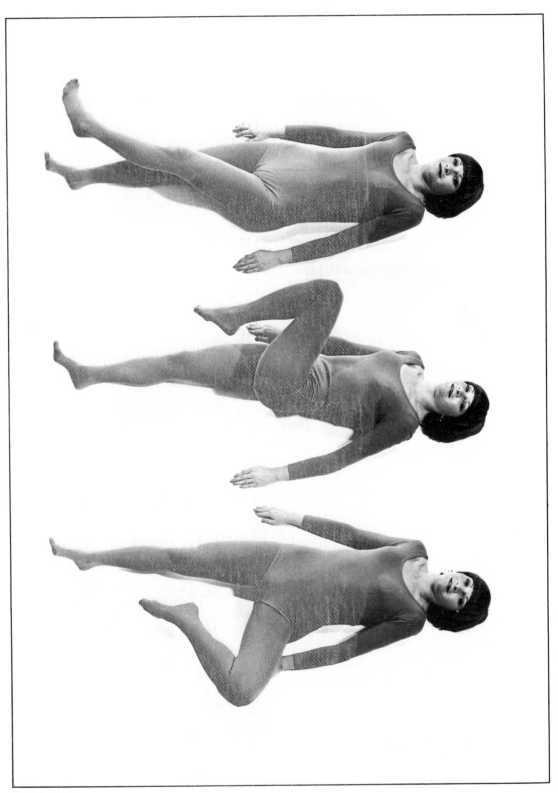

Leg Rotation

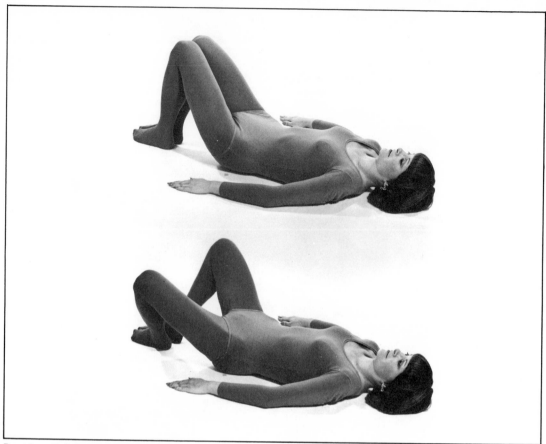

Bent Leg Fall Apart

B. COLLAPSING DRILLS

These drills are designed to promote the feeling of "letting go" – of consciously relaxing the muscles. They're called collapsing drills because that's precisely what they are: You should react as if you had been hit on the head with a blackjack. The holding force of your mind is suddenly eliminated, and you collapse. You should be aware of muscle tension, and then of a complete lack of tension. Make sure that your body and mind comprehend the distinction.

These drills can be done as a complete program, which will help to relax every key area of the body, or they can be excerpted and incorporated into your basic program.

 STRAIGHT LEG FALL APART

Lie on your back with your legs straight. Take a deep breath and hold it. Press your ankles and knees together lightly, and tighten your stomach muscles just enough to feel the tension. Hold for 3 seconds. Exhale slowly, letting the legs fall apart and the stomach muscles relax. Lie limply for 10 seconds. Repeat 8 times.

 BENT LEG FALL APART

Lie on your back with knees bent. While inhaling, press knees and ankles together lightly and hold for 3 seconds. Exhale, letting your legs fall apart. Relax for 10 seconds. Repeat 10 times.

ABDOMINAL TENSE AND RELAX

Lie on your back. While inhaling, puff up your stomach and hold for 3 seconds. Feel the tension with your finger tips. Now exhale and let your stomach muscles go limp. Remain limp for 5 seconds. Repeat 8 times.

 HIP LIFT AND RELAX

Lie on back with arms at sides. Take a deep breath and elevate your hips until they are just clear of the floor. Hold for 3 seconds, then exhale and let your hips drop. Repeat 8 times.

 ARM LIFT AND RELAX

Lie on your back with your hands a couple of feet out from your hips, arms straight. Take a deep breath, lifting your arms until they are just off the floor and hold for 3 seconds. Exhale and let them collapse. Repeat 6 times.

 HEAD LIFT AND RELAX

Lie on your back on bed or sofa. Breathing deeply, raise your head and upper back a few inches. Exhale and collapse. Repeat 6 times.

 BACK ARCH AND COLLAPSE

Lie on your back. Take a deep breath and elevate your chest and stomach until there is a good arch to your spine. Hold for a second or two, then collapse. Lie quietly for 5 seconds, feeling the relaxation of your muscles. Repeat 8 times.

 LATERAL HEAD COLLAPSE

Lie on your back. Take a deep breath and hold for a few seconds. As you exhale, let your head fall to one side. Repeat 6 times each side, trying to let the head collapse a little more loosely each time.

 ALLOVER COLLAPSE

Lie on your back and take a deep breath. Press your ankles and knees together, tense your stomach muscles slightly, raise your arms a few inches, lift your head a bit, and arch your back. Hold for a second or two, then exhale and collapse. Sink down as if all your energy had completely evaporated. Repeat 6 times.

C. BREATHING

Once you learn to associate relaxation with your breathing, you will have a skill that will help you in any moment of crisis. We all tend to breathe shallowly in a tense situation. Deep-breathing drills help to ease the "hollow feeling" in the pit of your stomach that usually means the muscles there have tightened up. You often see television performers, politicians, and others who are preparing to address an audience do this sort of drill. It's particularly important for them because tension in the muscles which control breathing can make them appear rushed, out of breath and nervous, spoiling the easy flow of words.

Lie on your back and begin to breathe slowly and deeply from the *stomach* (Many people breathe shallowly from the chest only). As you inhale, let your stomach puff up and as you exhale let it collapse. Do this 9 or 10 times with a steady, slow, and easy rhythm. Now repeat another 9 to 10 times, concentrating on allowing your whole body to go as limp and loose as possible every time you exhale. *Do not tense up first.* Rest a few seconds and repeat.

If you had to select only one relaxation routine, this "let go" breathing drill would be it. The relationship between breathing and relaxation is direct and strong. If you are especially tense, you should use this drill at intervals during the day, particularly when you are heading into or recovering from a high-anxiety situation. Remember to breathe from the stomach, inhaling and exhaling slowly and letting everything go loose and easy on the exhalation. Every exhalation should produce additional looseness; close your eyes and picture the muscles becoming slack so that tension seeps away.

Although it's best to lie down when you do the drill, you can do it at your desk, while watching television, or when you're reading. Make it a habit.

Step 4 – a Basic Program

The drills outlined so far will provide you with a basic relaxation program. If you do not have the time to do the full program, you can develop your own, shorter version using 2 or 3 exercises from each section, including the let-go breathing.

You should also draw on the exercises in Chapter 5 which are indexed under "Relaxation Control". These will add variety and refine your control over tension.

Step 5 – Daily Practice

The next step is to learn how to use your new skills during the daily moments of anxiety that inevitably arise. You will have to pay attention to your breathing and to developing that relaxation reflex. Relaxation will not come automatically until your skills have been tried under the "game conditions" of day-to-day living.

WORRY

Worry creates tension; fortunately, it can be eased by relaxation. Make sure that what you're worrying about is worth the time and effort. Sometimes, if you examine the problem carefully and logically, it goes away. Let's assume you've really got a problem and worry is the only way you can solve it (you think!).

First, take some time out, and do one or all of the basic relaxation drills. Is worry creating

buttterflies in your stomach? Do an extra drill or two for the stomach area – you can use those listed in the "Fitness at Work" chapter too.

The following eye exercise is also excellent, no matter what area of the body is tense. It's difficult to worry if your eyes are relaxed.

Inhale and at the same time close your eyes and squint a little – tighten up just enough to feel it. Hold for a couple of seconds, then exhale; relax, and try to let your eyeballs drop out onto your cheekbones. Repeat a few times. Again, make sure your mind is aware of the difference between tension and relaxation in the eye area.

These relaxation drills should help you get through your worry sessions. Even if they don't banish worry, at the very least they'll help to prevent the accompanying tension from doing physical damage – an important factor for the chronic worrier.

FEAR

Anticipation produces fear. Trips to the doctor or dentist, school examinations, speeches, interviews, important business meetings, championship games, thinking about the potential outcome of an activity or personal situation creates tension. The body responds to the mental stimulus or stress by producing the physical changes which were described earlier in this chapter. It does not take into account that the situation to which it is reacting may take place much later in the day, or tomorrow or even a couple of days later. It reacts *now*. Because for all intents and purposes your advance mental activity (worry) is the danger situation itself, there is a gathering of muscles and increased activity in the glandular system. If some sort of action does not follow immediately, this tension and its manifestations will not be released, nor will the chemical by-products disperse. Feeling tense, in turn, aggravates your fears.

If your stress situation involves an active situation, such as a speech or a game or an exam, keep your mind on *what* you are going to do, rather than on *how* well you are going to do. Thinking about the actual technical details helps to keep your mind off possible failure and reduces the stress response. Try to concentrate on something specific.

There is another method that some people have found helpful. One of Canada's top divers used to have severe pre-competition nerves. Don Webb, her coach, used a trick he called "nervous time". This athlete was encouraged to deliberately face her problem. She would say to herself: "OK, it's nervous time, my palms are wet, my mouth's dry, my heart's pounding. Let's get nervous." For her, this was much better than worrying about being nervous and scared; she was able to analyze her tension and control it.

This technique, of course, is not a panacea for all tension, but by making it less mysterious, it makes it less frightening. Often, if you hold up your particular demon by the scruff of the neck and dare it to do its worst, it simply fades away.

A third solution is to keep busy. If your fear/tension response starts a day or two in advance of the event, go to a show, read a book, go for a walk with a friend, listen to music. Do something you enjoy rather than sitting around and fussing.

If you have trouble sleeping, get up and do something rather than tossing and turning and worrying about the effects your loss of sleep is going to have on your performance. One night without sleep isn't going to reduce your mental and physical capabilities by an appreciable amount unless you let the worrying about it affect you. Too many people build a sleepless night into an insurmountable handicap—and *that's* what does them in. Negative thoughts produce negative performance.

Fourth, whenever you get the chance, run through the basic relaxation program. Concentrate on the let-go breathing drill.

Finally, even if you feel negative about your impending crisis, put on an act. Pretend to yourself and particularly to others that you are cheerful and optimistic. It will help you feel that way. Psychologists call your pre-event attitudes "self-fulfilling prophecies". If you think you are going to do badly, you will; if you think you are going to do well, you will. Learn to be positive and prophesy success.

NOISE, TURMOIL, ARGUMENTS

Life, to quote Shakespeare, is full of sound and fury. Children play at the top of their voices, people shout and disagree, construction crews rip up streets and tear down buildings, the neighbors' stereo blares. Sometimes we wonder how we can keep functioning with all that racket. Researchers have found that noise levels are a stressor which can affect health as well as hearing.

The best way to handle this kind of tension is to beat it before it starts. Work at becoming so generally relaxed that you are immune to the initial irritations which soon develop into major tension problems. Use the relaxation drills regularly, especially when you feel the noise and turmoil getting to you. The body, through its biofeedback mechanisms, will soon learn that the proper response to noise is relaxation, not tension.

TENSION AT WORK

Much of our tension stems from our jobs. We're frequently called on to do things we don't like, and to do them too fast or too long, at someone else's bidding. Sedentary jobs provide no release for the tension that builds up, be it from deadlines or sheer mechanical inefficiency and fatigue. We sit with shoulders and neck tensed up, hands clenched, teeth pressed together.

These tensions can be serious. They produce ulcers, high blood pressure, headaches and a host of other symptoms. That's why a whole chapter has been devoted to the subject of fitness and tension at work.

HOSTILITY

Hostility toward people, things, and situations is a sign of tension. It is also self-propagating: Tension creates hostility,

hostility creates more tension. Relaxation helps to break this vicious circle. A positive attitude is vital as well, so examine your mental as well as physical responses.

CRITICAL ATTITUDE

A team of doctors was asked by a group of business executives to find a way to alleviate tension. The doctors studied the problem and recommended that the businessmen learn the art of relaxation. They also suggested that their single most important cause of tension was a critical attitude. The doctors' investigations showed that the person who is especially critical of other people, situations, or conditions is under stress. Their advice: analyze but don't criticize; correct, but don't destroy; be tolerant and develop understanding.

FRUSTRATION

We all have to learn to deal with a daily routine of frustrations—from petty ones like doing without buttered toast in the morning because someone forgot to go to the store, to bigger ones like doing things the boss's way rather than your own, to even greater ones involving careers, marriage, and the whole course of our lives. These frustrations are all stressors. They create tension.

What can we do about them? We can learn to live with our frustrations by developing a philosophical attitude. This may involve self-examination and changing of outlook. More immediately, we can prevent frustration from interfering with health and physical efficiency by learning the technique of relaxation.

One immediate way of releasing frustration is to get what's bothering you off your chest. Unfortunately, all too often we get it off our chest by unloading it on someone else. We shout at wife or husband because the boss gave us a hassle; we shout at the telephone operator because somebody cut us off on the expressway.

Blowups are a safety valve, nature's way of releasing some of those inner tensions. But tension vented on someone else is usually returned in one form or another. Best to blow up in private. Find a place where you can really let go: shout, sing, scream, kick a pillow around the room. You can open an upstairs window and shout at the world if you like. (Just make sure that the neighbors aren't going to shout back.) Then do your relaxation program.

INACTIVITY

Almost all forms of exercise will help you get rid of some tension. That's why regular physical activity, even if it's simply walking, is a must for anyone with tension problems. Especially valuable is exercise that you enjoy, perhaps tennis, swimming, badminton, or skiing. However, if you're a highly competitive individual, be careful: You may be developing tensions through the drive to win or anger over making poor shots! Exercise, in this case, becomes a form of stress rather than a release. Continue with golf or tennis if you will, but seriously consider a non-competitive supplementary activity, such as hiking, dancing, or jogging to wind down tension levels.

Homo sapiens evolved as an active animal. When we cease activity, our bodies deteriorate and our anxieties, worries, and stresses multiply. Activity is essential to well-being.

MEDICAL FACTORS

If you are suffering from general tension and anxiety, and exercise and relaxation drills fail to help, the cause may be medical.

A thorough medical examination should always be the first step in any campaign to eliminate tension or to develop physical fitness. Talk over your plans with your physician, and discuss with him any particular points you may be wondering about.

You could be in a stress situation which your adaptation energy is incapable of handling and in danger of becoming a target for certain physical disabilities. Perhaps you should give serious thought to a change of life style: Flight, rather than fight, may be the answer.

NUTRITION

Poor nutrition is often the cause of tension, particularly if the diet is lacking in calcium, iron, the B complex and D vitamins, all of which relate to a strong, healthy nervous system. Chapter 7, Nutrition, discusses the importance of healthy eating patterns.

POSTURE

Poor posture is a sure way to develop tension. The body is designed to function efficiently in a certain alignment. If part of it is out of kilter, the rest of the body tries to compensate and some muscles are thrown into tension because they must do jobs they were not designed to do. Physiologists are placing more and more importance on the vital role of good posture in fitness and health. Poor posture is considered a basic cause of malfunction of the back and of many of the vital organs, including the lungs, heart, and stomach.

Poor posture and poor muscle tone go hand in hand, and their constant companions are fatigue and irritability. You can't stand erect for long if your muscles are no longer strong enough and flexible enough to hold you there without effort. That's why an overall fitness campaign is so important if poor posture is one of your problems.

TIGHT HANDS

The hands are a key tension area. Keep them loose. Check how you hold your pen, how you grip the steering wheel, your tennis racquet, a book, or the telephone. No need to crush everything you lay your hands on.

UNBALANCED LIFE STYLE

Narrow interests and activities are likely to cause tension. Try to insert some balance and variety into your life: Widen your interests and activities.

MENTAL IMAGE

''As a man thinketh, so is he'', the Bible tells us. A helpful trick in your campaign to beat tension is creating the right mental image of yourself. Take time off, especially when preparing for some special event, to imagine yourself sailing through your activities loose and relaxed. Picture yourself often as a confident, relaxed individual and you will become one.

Such mental imagery will be particularly helpful last thing at night when you snuggle down in bed. You'll fall asleep easier and sleep better.

Most of the world's top athletes in high-skill events are now trained to use mental imagery not only as part of the learning process but in their immediate preparation for an event. A diver will visualize the dive he or she is about to do in all its phases, right from the approach to entry into the water. It is vital to the execution of that dive that the mental image be perfect all the way through, so the diver concentrates on seeing himself making every movement exactly as it should be made.

HARMONY AND LAUGHTER

When people laugh a lot, when they like each other and get along, tension is rarely a problem. How's your laughter index these days?

Conversely, if you learn to relax, you are more likely to laugh, and to enjoy people. Your laughline and lifeline are inextricably linked. Learn to stay loose and you'll live longer, laugh louder, and enjoy life a lot more.

Step 6—Teaching

Teaching relaxation techniques to another person will help to develop your own skill and understanding faster. The athlete who turns to coaching when his playing days are over begins to really understand all the components of his skill. Defining a technique for someone else is the best way of learning it yourself.

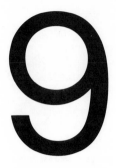

Fitness
at Work Too

FITNESS IS GOOD BUSINESS

Someday someone will feed into a big computer pertinent but at present imponderable information relating to fitness. The computer will then be programmed to find out three things:

1. Exactly how much money business and industry spend every year on absenteeism, medical care, hospitalization, and low productivity.

2. How closely these problems are related to the fitness of employees and executives.

3. What it would cost to invest in fitness programs to make sure that every employee and executive is fit enough to put in a full day's work at 100 per cent efficiency.

Tapes will roll, data will be processed, the machine will click or buzz or whatever big computers do – and you can be pretty certain that the answer will be heavily loaded in favor of fitness. More and more authorities are becoming convinced of its economic value.

Two of the leading authorities in the United States on disease resulting from physical inactivity – known as hypokinetic disease – are Drs. Wilhelm Raab and Hans Kraus. In their opinion:

"Unnecessary premature invalidism from orthopedic, cardiovascular and tension diseases is draining the economic resources of this country. Colossal sums are now being spent in connection with absenteeism, medical care, hospitalization and premature loss of earning power of workers and employees.

"If these detriments could be reduced, the expenses for preventive reconditioning programs would be dwarfed by the profits derived from them."[1]

Many firms have already begun to sense, dimly, that a penny saved is a penny earned. Embryonic fitness programs have been launched, some oriented to the executive rather than the person at the counter or machine. Unions have begun to press for fitness benefits to match those they receive in other areas of personal welfare. But so far it's only a drop in the bucket. Many countries in Europe are far ahead of North America in this field, and are reaping the benefits.

West Germany, for example, launched a network of reconditioning centers in 1955, operated jointly by insurance organizations and big industrial groups. Any worker whose fitness levels have fallen dangerously low (in an assessment by his insurance physician) has by law the right to be sent to such a center for up to four weeks. It doesn't cost him a cent, and it doesn't cut into his holiday period.

Among the symptoms which are considered cause for admission to the rehabilitation center are: fatigue which remains unrelieved by sleep; general nervous irritability; decrease of initiative and work efficiency; insomnia; feelings of frustration and despondency; abnormally high or low blood pressure; shortness of breath or angina-like chest sensations; muscular weakness; overweight.

The cost of maintaining and staffing such centers is huge, but they've proven their value: surveys have shown a 70 per cent decrease in lost working time. The cost of reconditioning a pre-invalid worker is only a fraction of the cost of training a substitute, and the postponement of invalidism and pension payments more than compensates for the four-week reconditioning period. Further, the maintenance cost of a bed in a reconditioning center is three or four times less than that of one in a hospital.

But the best time to start reconditioning is before the individual reaches a state of disrepair. And what better place to start than at the office? Everybody benefits.

The executive may scoff. What business is it of industry if the worker chooses to let himself go to pot? But evidence is piling up that it's *good* business which can be measured in dollars and cents.

Here are some examples:

● Dr. B. J. Geddes of Brigham Young University demonstrated that when exercise preceded tests involving memory, observation, concentration, and decisional efficiency, better scores were achieved.

● Sedentary workers, sitting for hours, have high rates of absenteeism, poor productivity, and dissatisfaction with their jobs.

● Studies of the physical and psychological needs of astronauts in flight established that regular periods of exercise eliminated a tendency toward decreased mental efficiency as well as making an absolutely essential contribution to their general health and fitness levels.

● At any given time the brain requires 15 per cent of the total oxygen available to the body in order to function efficiently. Inactivity contributes to decreased circulatory vigor and poorer extraction of oxygen from the air at the lungs. Less oxygen is distributed, and so the brain – our internal computer – goes on short rations.

If you live in a city or town, you probably spend at least eight hours (and frequently more) a day, five days a week, at your job. You take from 15 minutes to an hour to get to work, and chances are that you ride rather than walking or cycling. Your job requires you to be fairly inactive at a desk, or to stand at a counter or assembly line where you may indulge in mild upper body activity. In short, you are probably what is known as a sedentary worker.

This means you will be vulnerable to most of the following:

1. Degenerative diseases caused by inactivity.

2. Pooling of blood in the legs.

3. Stress, anxiety, and tension caused by deadlines, pressure to work fast, traffic / transportation frustrations.

4. Gradual loss of flexibility in certain muscle groups, particularly the hamstrings and chest.

5. Gradual loss of strength and tone of certain muscle groups, particularly the spinal, stomach, and leg muscles.

6. Decreased heart-wind-circulatory performance.

All of these problems will be compounded if you plop down in front of a television set when you get home – as most people do. We have truly become Homo Sedentarius. If Homo Habilis (tool-using man) was the beginning of civilization as we know it, surely Homo Sedentarius is the end.

If physical capability relates to work efficiency and enjoyment – and there is an increasing body of evidence that the link is a direct one – then industrialized western society has a serious problem.

The large corporations are beginning to realize this. But while you're waiting for management and boards of directors to get off their corporate gluteals, there's a lot the individual executive, office worker, or production-line employee can do at the personal level. Even if you don't feel like launching a full-scale personal fitness program, there are ways of beating tension, repairing muscle sag, and stopping the general physical deterioration which may be handicapping your chances for advancement and leaving you so worn out at the end of the day that you have little energy left for more than television. There are exercises that can be done right at the desk or during a coffee break and they only take a few minutes.

STRESS, TENSION, ANXIETY

Stress, tension, and anxiety are closely linked and together form the greatest single blockade against working efficiently and feeling good. They affect judgment, morale, enthusiasm, and thinking ability. They create fatigue, head and other bodily aches, and frustrations and irritations with others and with one's job. They can leave you exhausted at the end of the day with little zest for the evening's activities. Tension and anxiety can become residual. If there is no physical release, they can affect your sleep and your health. We've already talked about tension in Chapter 8, but a brief review will be useful here.

There are three principal sources of tension.

One is physiological. For example, sitting or standing for a long time in a constrained position can cause tension. Similarly, excessive muscle involvement in performing a task may result in "coordination tension"

The remaining sources of tension stem from emotional and mental factors and are described as psychological or affective tension. When this is expressed by the muscles the result is the same as coordination tension: soreness and stiffness of the areas involved, fatigue, and headaches. When you are under pressure (perhaps in a rush to get things done to meet a deadline), the nerves stimulating the muscles which are involved become overactive, producing excessive muscular contractions.

Without physical release, these tight muscles will not relax properly and you remain tense and possibly anxious for some time afterwards – the legacy of your mental stress.

Each individual is affected by tension in different parts of the body, depending on personality, posture, and the work being done. People working at a desk or a bench job which requires them to use their hands and arms are particularly prone to tension in the neck and shoulder area. Without realizing it, they gradually raise their shoulders higher and higher as they work; the hands grow tighter; and the neck, jaws, and facial muscles become rigid.

Affective tension can be blamed on poor posture habits – sitting too rigidly, for example, or slumping forward over your work. In the unexercised person slumping gradually produces weakened muscles in the back and neck, and shortened muscles in the chest. The lungs and other organs become cramped, the breathing is shallow, and the holding muscles of the upper body can no longer do their job properly. A permanent kyphosis, hump-back, may result.

On the other hand, consciously squaring your shoulders, straightening your back and holding your head high may only build tension. A military posture is not natural and becomes uncomfortable to maintain for any length of time.

Tension Control

The real answer is to tone up and strengthen the muscles which hold you in place so that you can easily maintain good relaxed posture while you're working. Second, learn to recognize tension and develop a relaxation reflex. Third, use a chair that supports you and sit properly. The height should be adjustable so that you can sit in a natural, relaxed position no matter what the height of the desk. Sit back in the chair so that it supports the lower back and hips and keep your feet flat on the floor – winding them around the legs of the chair creates tension. The spine should be straight but not rigid, and, if you have to bend over, do so from the waist rather than simply slumping the upper body.

The following exercises are designed principally to relieve neck and shoulder tension. If done often enough during the day, they will have a mild toning up effect on the muscles in this area as well.

These exercises involve tensing and relaxing the muscles until you feel the difference between the two sensations and learn to consciously relax any muscle that has become tense (a principle which was discussed fully in Chapter 8). Eventually, in a sort of biofeedback spinoff, the muscles themselves will begin to sense the difference and develop a relaxation reflex.

ex HIGH STRETCH AND RELAX

Stand erect with feet comfortably apart, hands on head. *Slowly* straighten your arms overhead, stretching as high as you can. Hold maximum stretch for 5 seconds, then relax, on the exhale. Repeat 6 times.

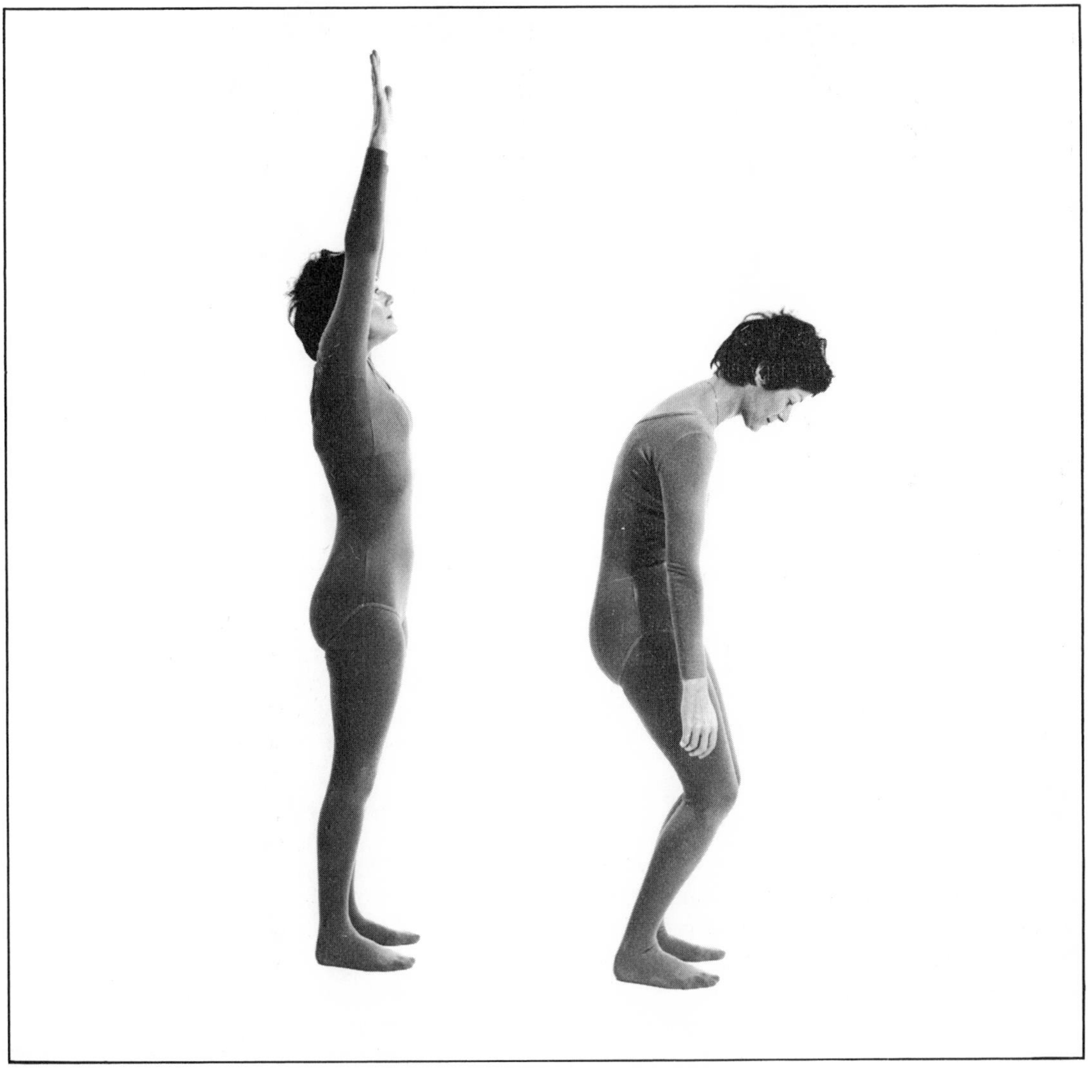

High Stretch and Relax

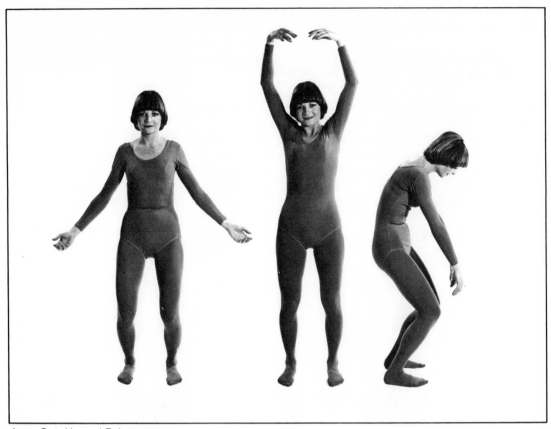

Arms Out, Up and Relax

 ARMS OUT, UP AND RELAX

Stand with feet comfortably apart. While inhaling, lift arms out to the sides and overhead, pulling your stomach in and lifting your chest high. Exhale and let the arms drop down limply at your sides, the knees go soft, and the chin drop to the chest. Repeat 6 times.

 LATERAL NECK STRETCH

Stretch your head slowly to one side while reaching down and away from you with the opposite arm. Hold stretch position for 5 seconds, then relax. Repeat 6 times to each side.

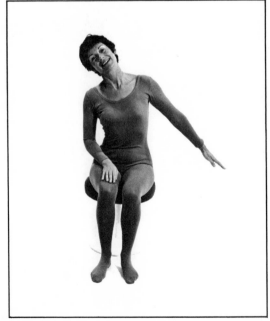

Lateral Neck Stretch

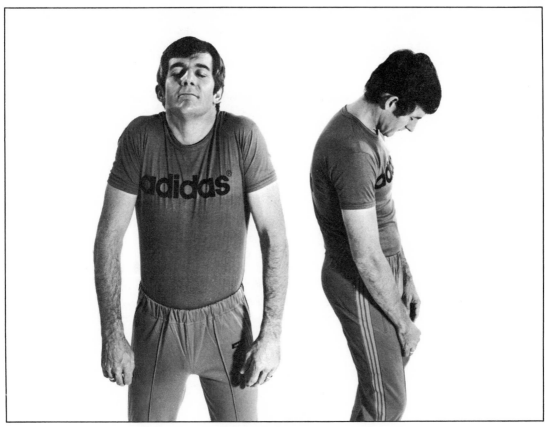

Shrugging

 SHRUGGING

With arms hanging at sides, draw your shoulders as high as you can on the inhale. Hold tension for 3 seconds, then exhale and relax. Repeat 6 times.

Stretching exercises should always be done slowly. If you move too fast, the muscles may react by tightening up slightly, the way they do when the doctor taps your knee with a little hammer to test your reflexes. This is called the myotatic reflex. The muscles respond to slow stretching by relaxing slightly in what is called the inverse myotatic reflex.

The above exercises relieve neck and shoulder tension. But tension hits other areas as well. Here are some desk exercises for the rest of the body which not only help to release tension but have a stimulating and refreshing effect by improving your circulation and by helping the blood stream carry oxygen to your muscles, brain, and organs.

 SEATED CALF STRETCH

Sitting in a chair, stretch one leg out in front of you as far as you can, leading with the heel and pulling the toes back toward your shin. Hold for 5 seconds and relax. Repeat 6 times with each leg.

CHEST STRETCH

In a seated position, lift and expand your chest using your muscles rather than your lungs. Hold 3 seconds, relax, and exhale. Repeat 6 times.

 ARM STRETCH

Stretch your arms out to your sides at shoulder height as far as possible. Hold 3 seconds, then let them drop loosely to your sides. Repeat 6 times.

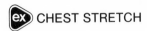 HEAD CIRCLING

In a sitting position, let your chin drop to your chest. Keeping the neck relaxed, rotate your head *slowly* in big circles, 6 times to each side. Allow your jaw to hang open loosely. Feel the stretching action on the muscles of the neck and back, and try to imagine the tension oozing out of them.

 SEATED TOE TOUCH

With your chair moved back from your desk, sit on the front edge with feet flat on the floor directly under your knees. Bend forward slowly, allowing your head to hang loosely, and slowly reach toward your toes. Stretch for 5 seconds, return to starting position and repeat 6 times.

 SEATED HEAD KNEE TOUCH

Sit on front of chair well away from desk. Clasp one leg behind the knee and lift it as high as you can toward your chest. Try to touch it with your head slowly, no sudden ducking of the head. Do 8 times with alternate legs.

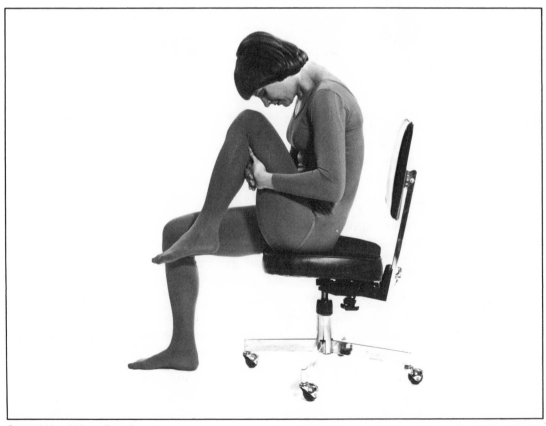

Seated Head Knee Touch

During all these exercises, the mind should be playing an active role. You should be trying to visualize the feelings of tension and relaxation, and learning to recognize them. It may help to say to yourself: "This is tension, this is how it feels," and "This is relaxation, this is how it feels, this is what I want."

Do these drills any time you feel tense and have a moment to spare. You can use any or all of them – a couple of neck and shoulder exercises if hard typing is beginning to tire you, or some leg stretching work if your calves are a bit cramped – whatever makes you feel good.

The full story of relaxation is presented in Chapter 8. If this brief program intrigues you, enlarge it by using the methods suggested there.

Traffic Jam

In 1973 the *British-American Medical Journal* published the results of a study done in London which linked tremendous increases in heart-circulatory problems to stress in heavy traffic – one more example of what tension can do: you're a wreck even before you arrive at your job!

One answer would be walking to work, but work and home frequently are separated by several miles. It is possible to leave the car or subway some distance from the office and hike the last couple of miles, thus avoiding the frustrations of downtown traffic and reaping the benefits of physical activity. A brisk walk can set you up for the day, and also release a lot of the built-up tension after work.

The weather, particularly in winter, may force you back under cover, either into your car or the subway. Too bad, because psychologists say that we unconsciously resent being confined. We react with some degree of frustration, and this frustration usually manifests itself in tension and/or anxiety.

Doing something physical is the best way to release these symptoms. When someone cuts you off at the light or takes your parking spot, you usually just sit there and seethe inside. The adrenal glands pump up the blood pressure, the heart rate rises, circulation and oxygen supply to the muscles are restricted by a reflex tensing of the muscles, and within seconds your system feels as if it's been squeezed through a wringer.

Chances are your whole morning's work output will be affected. What to do about it? Walking briskly the last couple of miles will help. But here's a program you can follow without even getting out of your car.

First, work on attitude – a positive philosophy. Think constructively about what you are going to do this week, the weekend's pleasure, the plans for your next vacation. Use every trick you know to get your mind off the traffic incident that's just sent your blood pressure soaring. Refuse to dwell on it. Remember that your feeling of being trapped in your little box is helping you to magnify it out of proportion.

Help yourself to relax by regulating your breathing. Tension spreads from the hands and the neck and shoulders down into your stomach and diaphragm, making your breathing shallow and rapid. You can reverse the process by slow, moderately-deep rhythmic breathing. When you exhale, concentrate on letting the whole body relax as you let the air go. This will make you more comfortable, while the slow rhythm will reduce the heart rate. Then exercise – get some tension-releasing physical activity.

"Exercise", you ask, "in a moving car?"

No, not in a moving car. But when you're locked in a traffic jam or stopped at a light, there are certain things you can do to persuade the muscles to unlock and let the blood flow again. Here's a check list.

HANDS

Are your knuckles white and the fingers locked on the wheel? Loosen up. Stretch the fingers, shake your hands, twist the wrists. Then lower them into your lap. Using a continuous raised-arm driving position can elevate blood pressure slightly. In normal traffic, holding the top half of the wheel is best for control, but in slow-moving jam-ups, you can safely drop your hands to the lower half of the wheel so they are below heart level. When you move off, check your finger pressure on the wheel every so often. Don't strangle it.

SHOULDERS

Shrug your shoulders up toward your ears, hold for a few seconds and let them drop loosely down. People who develop headaches while driving often have problems with neck and shoulder tension.

NECK

Rotate the head slowly a couple of times, first to the left, then to the right. Let the jaw drop so that the muscles are loose and relaxed.

STOMACH

Butterflies in the stomach? Anxiety about a crisis day often causes stomach tension which is aggravated by the first traffic jam. Pull the stomach in and up, hold for a few seconds, then let it relax. Repeat.

PELVIC AREA

Press your knees together for a few seconds moderately hard, then relax and let them fall apart. Repeat.

LEGS

Twisting the ankle to stretch the calf muscles, tensing and relaxing the calf muscles, flexing the toes, are all useful activities which can be done in the car.

POSTURE

Hunching over the wheel will cramp the chest and interfere with breathing. Sit erect comfortably. Adjust the seat so that your knees are slightly flexed and higher than the hips – if you have to reach with outstretched legs for the accelerator, the lower back will be under stress.

KEEPING FIT

Exercise through the working day can help you to function better in your job, and to enjoy your recreation after work. If you can stimulate circulation just before a work assignment or the moment when a key decision must be made, so much the better.

The activity need not be long or particularly vigorous, if it is repeated frequently. Do one or two exercises at a time, whenever you get the chance. Apart from the immediate benefits, they'll raise your general fitness level to a surprising degree when done regularly for a few weeks.

A complete and fully effective rebuilding job cannot be done, however, unless you are prepared to undertake a comprehensive fitness campaign utilizing the principles and exercises described in Chapters 3, 4, and 5.

Flexibility

Bending over a desk or bench all day interferes with proper breathing. Some cardiologists believe poor posture and lack of chest flexibility put stress on the heart-circulatory system.

When the chest wall remains in a concave position long enough, the muscles, especially the intercostal muscles between the ribs begin to lose their ability to function. Tension develops. Breathing and circulation are impaired.

While there are other areas which lose flexibility if you are sedentary day after day, none is quite so important to your well-being as the chest area. Do the following three exercises whenever you get a chance: at your desk, in your car, or at home while you're watching television.

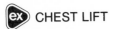

CHEST LIFT

Lift the chest wall out and up as high as you can, arching your back and moving your head backwards. Hold for a few seconds and relax. Repeat.

 ## LATERAL CHEST STRETCH

Sit erect with your chest held high. Bend sideways as far as you can and hold for several seconds. Now bend to the opposite side. Repeat 7 to 8 times.

 ## CHEST LIFT REPETITION

Do the chest lift as before, but instead of holding the stretch position, pause for only a second. Repeat 10 times in a series of rhythmic movements, rest 15 seconds, and repeat.

Oxygen Transport

A vigorous circulation which carries oxygen to all parts of the body is just as important to you as it is to the athlete. It gives you the stamina to carry on without loss of functional efficiency. When you're concentrating and thinking hard, the brain may utilize up to 50 per cent of the body's total oxygen supply. If that supply is restricted, the brain will be robbed of "fuel".

The cerebral athlete has little opportunity to exercise his heart and lungs; consequently, they deteriorate quickly (you start to puff after going up only a few stairs at a moderate pace). The body runs out of oxygen very quickly because it is no longer efficient in extracting it from the air in the lungs, and getting it into the muscles. You go into "oxygen debt" just the way you go into financial debt when you haven't enough money in the bank.

If you smoke, the following exercises are even more important. Smokers generally have a lower oxygen uptake than non-smokers; they can improve it at almost the same rate, however.

 ## STOMACH PUMPING

Sit comfortably. Alternately pull in your stomach and puff it out with a pumping action for 10 to 15 seconds at a brisk rate. Rest 15 seconds and repeat. This exercise helps to distribute the reserves of blood which are stored in the stomach area and also to tone up the muscles. It can be done almost any time you happen to think of it – at your desk, while watching television, or in your car while waiting for a stoplight.

 ## QUARTER SQUAT

Stand beside your desk and do 25 or 30 quarter squats at a brisk pace. Quarter squats are just what they imply – go down only a quarter of the way. Full squats are not advisable because of a possible adverse effect on knee ligaments.

 ## WALKING

Get up from your desk and walk about briskly for 2 to 3 minutes using a vigorous arm action, or stand beside your desk and walk on the spot for 2 or 3 minutes at moderate tempo, lifting the knees to stomach height.

 ## JOGGING ON THE SPOT

Do a stationary jog beside your desk for 1 or 2 minutes. Emphasize the knee action.

 ## SHOULDER SHRUG

Sit or stand comfortably. Shrug your shoulders up toward your ears, then drop them down as low as you can. Continue this action at a brisk rhythm for 30 seconds.

STATIONARY CRAWL

Sit relaxed. Move your arms and shoulders in a simulated-crawl swimming action at a moderate tempo for a minute or two.

 ## LATERAL SIDE BEND

Sit relaxed. Bend your upper body from side to side at a fairly quick tempo for 30 seconds.

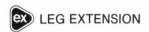 LEG EXTENSION

Sit relaxed far enough from your desk to allow full leg movement. Extend first one leg and then the other in front of you at a brisk pace for a minute or two.

Feet, Legs, Back

The muscles of the legs are designed to work as peripheral pumps which help the heart shift blood back from the nether regions of the body. People who stand at their work — sales clerks, machine operators, production line operators, barbers — may have a problem: their "leg pumps" become inactive. Blood collects, forcing the heart to work harder to distribute the remaining supply to other parts of the body, including the brain.

To prevent circulatory problems, walk back and forth whenever possible; do a few half squats; get some leg exercise during coffee breaks and lunch, and take a few minutes to lie with the feet higher than the rest of the body. This helps the heart to counter the force of gravity and pump the "pooled" blood out of the legs.

When you get home, put your feet up when you're reading the paper or watching television. If your legs ache, massage them with a wet towel in which you have wrapped some ice, starting from the feet and working upwards.

Gravity is the culprit in another difficulty which affects many standing workers: low back pain. It may be linked to disc problems or may be caused by weak stomach muscles which allow the pelvis to tilt forward, throwing a strain on the lower back.

As an example of how potent the pull of gravity can be, one research project showed that some standing workers were actually shorter at the end of the day than they were in the morning.

If you have trouble with low back pain, see a doctor. If he assures you that there is no disc involvement, the answer is strengthening exercises for the stomach and back. (See those listed in Chapter 5.)

You can get temporary relief by standing with one foot on a low stool. Make sure, however, that you alternate feet from time to time so that you do not induce a sideways curvature of the spine by having one foot higher than the other. Good standing posture is also important. Many people stand back on their heels with their pelvis thrust forward — a sure way to place an extra strain on the lower back.

If you have to deal with frustrating or tension-producing situations in your job or do difficult precision work, neck and shoulder tension may also affect you. Do the exercises suggested earlier in this chapter and study the chapter on relaxation.

If your arches are creating problems, use the special foot exercises outlined in Chapter 5 to strengthen them.

Meals and Coffee Breaks

The food you eat in the morning is the fuel your body uses until lunch. There are a number of research projects which show that people who rush in to work or school after only a cup of coffee have far less stamina, concentration, and mental capacity than those who have eaten a good breakfast. They are also subject to increased anxiety and irritability — the body and the brain are crying out for fuel to keep them going.

The answer some people choose is frequent coffee breaks. They crave sugar in the form of candy and sweet drinks. But in this context sugar is not really an "energy food" and actually compounds the problem.

Refined sugar is a powerful stimulant which causes the vital organs to work harder and faster, with an explosive effect on the digestive system. It produces a quick pickup — followed by just as quick a slump. As glucose rushes to the bloodstream, the pancreas starts to produce insulin to get rid of it because too much sugar in the blood can cause diabetic symptoms.

Because of the extra insulin produced, the pendulum swings the other way, and you have even less sugar in the bloodstream than when you started (not to mention added deposits in the fat cells).

The brain requires sugar in the bloodstream in order to absorb oxygen, its primary fuel. When cheated of its "fuel", the brain produces symptoms that can range from vague feelings of nervousness, to anxiety, restlessness, confusion, lack of concentration, memory loss, and even chronic fatigue.

More important, the high and low blood sugar extremes caused by eating and drinking too many sugar-containing foods can lead to a faulty metabolism. The pancreas starts producing too much or too little insulin. Too little insulin produces symptoms of diabetes and possibly even diabetes itself, while too much results in "hypoglycemia" or not enough sugar in the blood. The most noticeable symptom of hypoglycemia is an unusually strong craving for sweets: the body is improperly metabolizing sugar and other carbohydrates.

And that's why instead of helping, your coffee break may be contributing to your problems.

This is a good point to remember if you're going on a long drive, especially at night. Eating too many sweets may make you drowsy. Make sure your pre-departure meal includes sufficient protein, and include proteins in any snack you take en route. Coffee with sugar may hamper rather than help your efforts to stay awake.

Unlike sugar and candy, protein foods provide a slow, steady source of glucose, thus avoiding an insulin reaction.

A good balanced breakfast with protein foods helps you to keep "fueled up" throughout the morning. You think more clearly, suffer less from anxiety and fatigue, and have less craving for fat-producing snacks or heavily-sweetened tea or coffee.

When you go on your coffee break, take a wedge of cheese or some nuts and a glass of milk instead of a soft drink, Danish pastry, or piece of pie. Protein-rich snacks provide the gradually-released blood sugar you need through the rest of the morning, and may also help you cut down on the size of your lunch. A big lunch – which you may feel like eating if you've avoided breakfast and stoked up on sugar foods instead – throws a load on the digestive system which must process all that food. Digestion draws heavily on the body's blood supply, and so you head back to work feeling lethargic and heavy, with the brain still crying out for oxygen in order to cope with the afternoon's workload.

Caffeine usually is regarded as the culprit which does the damage in coffee and, to a lesser extent, in tea. But it is obvious that sugar can be a problem as well, particularly for those who drink a lot of these beverages (which also contain certain oils which are harmful in excess). So, while coffee and tea may temporarily relieve feelings of fatigue and depression, they may also intensify anxieties, keep you awake at night, and raise your blood pressure. Coffee in particular has been implicated in gastritis, certain heart and artery disorders and, by stimulating the action of the kidneys, can cause some vitamins and minerals to be passed through the intestines before they are properly absorbed.

Certain people, apparently, are more susceptible to the effects of coffee and tea than others. Some tend to turn them into crutches to prop up flagging spirits or to relieve boredom, drinking 20, 30, or more cups per day.

Drinking de-caffeinated coffee may not solve the problem, because the sugar and oils remain. Try to cut back your coffee consumption to half a dozen cups a day, or less.

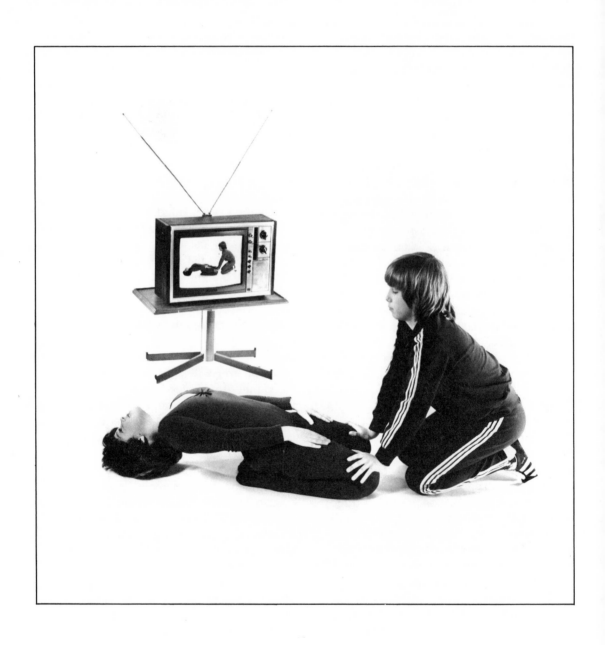

Fitness for Children

10

Start Them Young

THE FORMATIVE YEARS

When several hundred Toronto children aged 6 to 12 were tested for general muscle strength, arm strength, flexibility, balance, and coordination, 85 per cent of these youngsters were unable to achieve what were considered minimum passing grades. They were particularly inept in leg flexibility, arm strength and general motor ability, muscle sense, and coordination. The cross-Canada picture was the same.

The situation is not improving. Schools are noting an increasing deficiency in basic motor ability and muscle development in children, particularly in those growing up in large apartment blocks whose parents use television as a pacifier or baby sitter. When television first became a mass medium in the early 50s, an entirely new breed of child was spawned – underexercised, overfed, and uninvolved. At the same time, compulsory physical education began to disappear from the school curriculum.

This child is now an adult. Statistics show that he or she is likely to have a heart attack at a far earlier age than ever before, is prone to degenerative diseases, is overweight, suffers from emotional problems such as anxiety and tension, and is still uninvolved in regular physical activity. However, he or she now worries about the situation, and is a good market for fitness fads and books, especially those which promise short cuts and no-effort programs.

Unfortunately, many of these adults, without realizing it, are teaching their children to become physically inept as well. To quote former world swimming record holder Elaine Tanner: "I believe the love and desire to participate is handed down from one generation to another. Youngsters use their parents as a guideline."[1]

Most authorities agree that the first five years of a child's life are of particular importance in shaping attitudes. During these years, the child looks to the mother for approval or disapproval. It is she, more than the father who forms the child's positive attitudes toward physical activity, or avoidance of it. If she uses television as a means of control and repeatedly tells him or her to be quiet instead of participating in normal roughhouse play with other children, and if she is overprotective and overanxious, the child learns that active patterns of behavior are wrong.

Children fall, cut and burn themselves, and run risks of all kinds because they are inexperienced and naive. They must, of course, be protected from danger that threatens life and safety, but in the process of protection they must also be taught how to avoid such danger in the future. Nature provided for that by giving them bones which break easily and also mend easily, constitutions that are infected by and throw off illnesses, thereby achieving future immunity and minds that bounce back from trouble.

Some mothers are overly afraid that their child may fall, may suffer cuts and bruises, may "overdo" physical activity. Such mothers feed their child's fears with their own; the child learns that active, aggressive behavior is to be avoided. Climbing is dangerous. Running is bad because you may get exhausted. Wrestling with other children is antisocial. Give up the struggle. Sit quietly and be good!

Of such attitudes are physical incompetents born.

How are such children to get enough hard exercise to develop the big muscle masses in the legs, arms, and back? They need to run, climb, push, shove, and shout in the games their bodies demand for growth. It's more than a matter of letting off steam. The child is testing himself or herself, trying out new muscles and skills, developing coordination of mind and body, exploring fresh ideas and gaining self-assurance.

When the child enters elementary school, attitudes toward physical activity will be to some degree already established. The body's development will relate closely to such attitudes.

Children who have been cast in a role of passive dependence will find that their ability to handle the physical and mental stresses of the future has been jeopardized. Dozens of research projects point out children with posture defects, children with basic physiological weaknesses (both muscular and cardiovascular), children with serious emotional problems, children with passive attitudes toward physical activity, children

carrying too much fat — all increasing at a rate which alarms many authorities.

The elementary school years are almost as crucial to the child as the earlier ones. Having learned to use his muscles, he should now be learning to use them *well* to gain the fundamental skills and interests which lead to physical prowess in later years.

Physiologists agree that a strong physical foundation is best developed between the ages of 6 and 12. Unfortunately, there is evidence that this is not happening as efficiently as it should.

This is what the authoritative American publication, *Physical Fitness Research Digest*, had to say in its October 1973 issue:

"Orientation of boys and girls to the need for exercise as a way of life should be stressed in order to attain and maintain total effectiveness. Studies reported here and in earlier Digests have shown the totality of the individual: that physical, psychosocial and mental accomplishments are interrelated."[2]

Our doctors have provided us with protection against diseases caused by germs and viruses, but there is little social pressure to develop the physical capabilities needed to withstand the diseases of degeneration: heart trouble, arteriosclerosis, hypertension, slipped discs.

What Can You Do as a Parent?

First, examine your own attitudes to physical fitness and physical activity. Is your child likely to develop a positive approach to the development of his muscles and skills? If not, perhaps you should re-examine your role, which should start as soon as the child is old enough to respond to you.

Second, what shape is your child in? Does he/she have good posture, stamina, strength, flexibility, coordination? Starting at age 4, one way to find out for sure is to use the tests listed in Chapter 3. They'll be fun to do, and they'll tell you a lot about the capabilities of your youngster. If he or she scores below the halfway mark on any of the tests, you should start thinking seriously about a development program based on the information in this chapter.

Third, examine your child's posture. Common faults are illustrated later in this chapter. If you note serious deviations from the norm, start doing something about them. Research is uncovering vital links between poor posture and the physical ailments which afflict us as we get older. Preventive medicine *now* can save your child a lot of grief later.

Fourth, is your child interested in sports? Give some thought to channeling his or her interest into sports which have carry-over value outside of school. No need to take him out of hockey if he enjoys it, but if he also learns to enjoy skiing, tennis, or badminton now, he'll have a sport he can play for the rest of his life.

If your child does not enjoy sports, perhaps he is physically ill-equipped to handle them on equal footing with his peers. Encourage him in games within his capabilities, and get started on a program to build the strength, stamina, and coordination he needs to enjoy a more active future.

Fifth, what sort of physical education program does your child's school have? If it's little more than an afterthought, perhaps its time you had serious discussions with other parents about improving the situation. If the parents don't care, the schools may not care either — and they'll be teaching physical failure.

How Fit Is Fit Enough?

If you were absolutely positive of your child's destiny, this would be a relatively easy question to answer. A professional hockey player, for example, would need high levels of strength, endurance, flexibility, agility, and so on. But an artist would probably be wasting his time trying to develop bulging biceps and the capacity to run a mile in four minutes. Fitness is relative.

However, every child must attain a basic level of fitness in order to mature into a healthy, active adult. If the years between 6 and 12 are the most critical in the development of the body, what is your son or daughter building for the future?

Does he or she have:

1. Muscular strength to sustain proper posture; perform daily tasks without fatigue, meet special effort loads without excess stress and recover quickly from them; provide protection from strain and injury; participate well enough in group activities to enjoy them; sustain health of vital organs?

2. Flexibility to perform a full range of muscle and joint movements with ease; be free of muscle tension?

3. Endurance (stamina) to participate freely in effort-requiring activities without undue fatigue, and to recover quickly after hard effort?

4. Motor ability (agility and coordination) to participate in games and physical activities with reasonable enjoyment, skill, and safety?

5. Emotional and physical capacity for relaxation so that activities performed under stress can be maintained with reasonable freedom from stress symptoms; the ability to regain composure (relaxation) following such situations?

6. Freedom from important posture defects which could interfere with physical efficiency, comfort, health, and appearance?

7. Freedom from the hazards and restrictions of both overweight and underweight?

8. Sound nutrition so that the body is able to repair itself adequately and develop fully to its potential strength and size, and so that energy levels remain high?

9. Freedom from disease and health problems generally?

Research shows that not one in 100 Canadian youngsters can meet all these requirements.

Further, while the physical education programs now being presented by many schools are no longer capable of rectifying this situation, it's not entirely their fault. Parents frequently tell their children: "Do as I say", but the message the child responds to is: "Do as I do." So many parents are sedentary, it's no wonder the children are physically unfit.

Fitness Begins at Home

There are two solutions to the problem of the unfit child. First, use the program suggested here as a basis for fitness education for your children. Second, start a family fitness program in which your children are involved. The latter, of course, is the best way. It may be hard for the child to understand why he has to get fit when you are not. On the other hand, while you may not be prepared to become personally involved in such a project, there's no reason why you can't be the coach and inspire your "team" to a better performance. Physical activity need not be drudgery for a child. Make it a game. Generate interest, provide easily attainable objectives, measure progress, and above all, reward effort and achievement; you'll be surprised at how much enthusiasm you can arouse.

On the other hand, if you can make it a family project, the rewards will be more than doubled. Your own fitness levels will benefit, your family will be drawn closer together in seeking a common goal, and your children

will move toward an active life style. Physically and mentally, there's no better investment in the future.

Always remember that in projects of this sort children should be guided and encouraged, rather than driven and commanded. They are highly motivated to learn at this stage in their development, but if they are ordered to follow an exercise program which may not only seem dull but may be slightly beyond their capabilities, that motivation may soon fade or be channeled in another direction.

The goals they seek must be *their* goals, not yours alone. Testing and retesting are as important for children as they are for adults. They must be able to see their progress; they require objectives toward which this progress is taking them, and they should have lots of love and support en route.

The First Step: Testing

Testing and measurement is the starting point for any fitness program. The technique is described in Chapter 3.

Before you test your child, give him or her a pep talk. Make sure the child knows that he or she is to try as hard as possible, but that it is fun and there is nothing to fear from possible failure. Some youngsters may worry that you won't love them any more if they do badly, or that you'll make fun of them and tell them that Johnny Smith down the street could have scored much better. Make fitness a game from the start and eliminate the possibility that any weakness or failure will affect your relationship with your child. The child must know this. Trust and confidence are essential if the project is to become mutual and not just "something that daddy says I have to do". This means you must be careful not to show any signs of disappointment or discouragement if your child fails a test or does not progress quickly.

The child must not lose confidence. This does not mean that you can't be strict about regular routine and proper execution of workouts. But be aware that you are trying to create a positive life style rather than inflicting military discipline on somebody who may decide (secretly) that life is going to be much easier once conscription is over!

THE "BIG 7" – A BASIC FITNESS PROGRAM

The following exercises are designed to train and develop the basic physical needs of your child: strength, flexibility, and a certain amount of heart-wind conditioning for endurance. However, the importance of games involving running, jumping, and all-over body movement cannot be overemphasized in the total mental and physical development of youngsters. The child who comes home from school and immediately heads for the television set misses out on this vital area of the growth process.

While this basic exercise program will do an excellent job of developing an all-round fitness level, you would be wise to look closely at the testing results and incorporate into your child's program some of the exercises from Chapter 5 and from the "Specific Problems" section later in this chapter. These will help to develop agility, extra strength and stamina, and promote relaxation. They will be particularly useful if your child has a sports ambition. You should also study the section on posture, and make sure that your child is doing whatever remedial exercises may be necessary. The time to cure posture defects is when they are just starting, rather than when they are so ingrained that they are next to impossible to put right.

This program is suitable for both boys and girls, and children can start it as soon as they are old enough to understand your instructions. The younger they are, the easier it will be to instil regular exercise habits.

Before you start your child on the program, consider the following points:

1. Make sure each exercise is done exactly according to instructions and as illustrated. Stress the fact that the stomach should be held in during each exercise, and make sure that good posture is maintained when resting between exercises.

2. Praise the child after each exercise session. Point out progress and provide rewards from time to time.

3. Once a week have the child try for a record in one particular exercise. Select a different one each week.

4. It's a good idea to decide ahead of time how many days a week your child is going to work out, and make up a chart on which to keep track of progress. Mark new records with stars, and give special awards for progress and regularity of workouts. Provide incentives and make the drills fun, rather than a dull daily grind.

1. ALLOVER STRETCH

Start from a completed push-up position with the arms straight and hands directly under the shoulders. Lower hips as close as possible to the floor, pulling the head back as far as you can. Hold for 3 seconds. Then raise the buttocks as high as possible, pulling in the stomach and tucking the chin toward the chest while forcing the heels to the floor. Hold for 3 seconds. The arms remain straight at all times. If there is not enough strength to hold an extended push-up position, the knees instead of the feet may be used for support.

Reps: 6 to 10

Purpose: Tones major muscle groups.

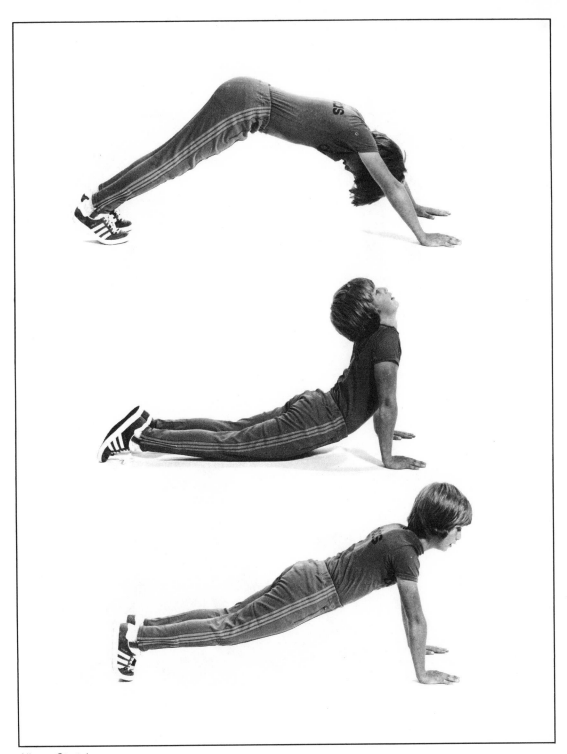

Allover Stretch

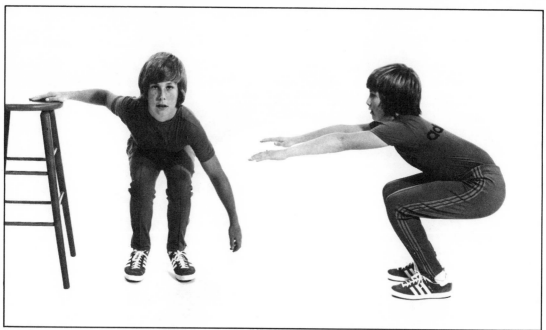

Half Squat

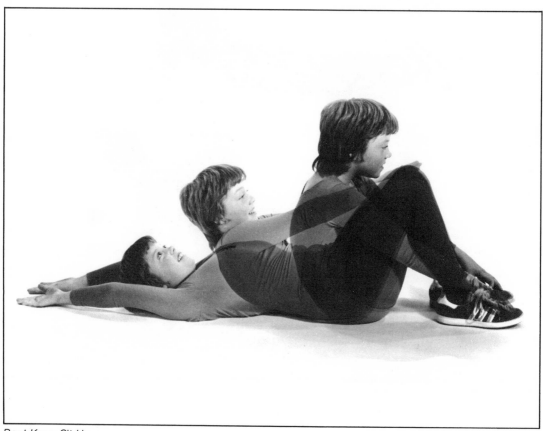

Bent Knee Sit Up

2. HALF SQUAT

Stand with arms extended in front and feet hip-width apart. Lower the hips as though sitting in a chair. The knees should remain hip-width apart. Stand up and repeat. If there is difficulty with balance, the hand can be used for support, resting lightly on a chair or table. See Chapter 5 for alternative methods.

> **Reps:** 3x6 to 3x20   **Rest:** 15 sec.
> **Purpose:** Develops strength and endurance in major muscles of the legs.

3. HIGH STRETCH AND RELAX

Stand with feet comfortably apart. Take a deep breath, pull in stomach and stretch arms as high as possible overhead. Hold for 3 seconds, then exhale, and relax. Allow the knees to bend slightly and repeat. If possible, this exercise should be done several times during the day, especially first thing on getting out of bed.

> **Reps:** 6 to 12
> **Purpose:** Overall stretch and relaxation.

4. BENT KNEE SIT UP

Lie on back with knees bent at right angles, arms stretched out overhead. Sit up, touching chest to knees and hands to toes. Relax and repeat in a quick, even rhythm. If an unaided sit up is not possible, the feet should be held or anchored.

> **Reps:** 3x6 to 3x20   **Rest:** 15 sec.
> **Purpose:** Develops abdominal strength and endurance.

5. PUSH-UP

Lie face down with hands on floor shoulder-width apart. Push upwards, keeping the body and legs straight, until the arms are fully extended. Then lower the body until chest and chin touch floor. Repeat. The stomach and knees must not touch the floor.

If there is insufficient strength to do a full push-up, there are two alternatives. One is to use the knees for support instead of the toes while pushing upward. The second alternative is to start from the completed push-up position, slowly lowering the body to the floor. Then use the knees to aid arm extension, and again lower the body. Test regularly, and as strength improves, gradually incorporate full push-ups into the exercise. See Chapter 5 for variations of the push-up.

> **Reps:** 3x4 to 3x20   **Rest:** 15 sec.
> **Purpose:** Develops strength and endurance in arms, shoulders, and upper body.

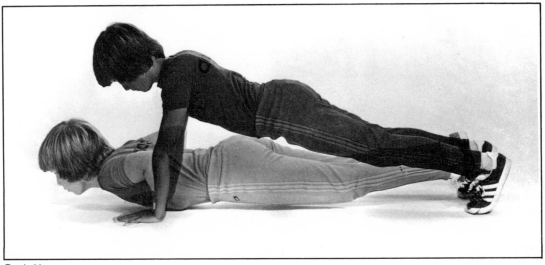

Push-Up

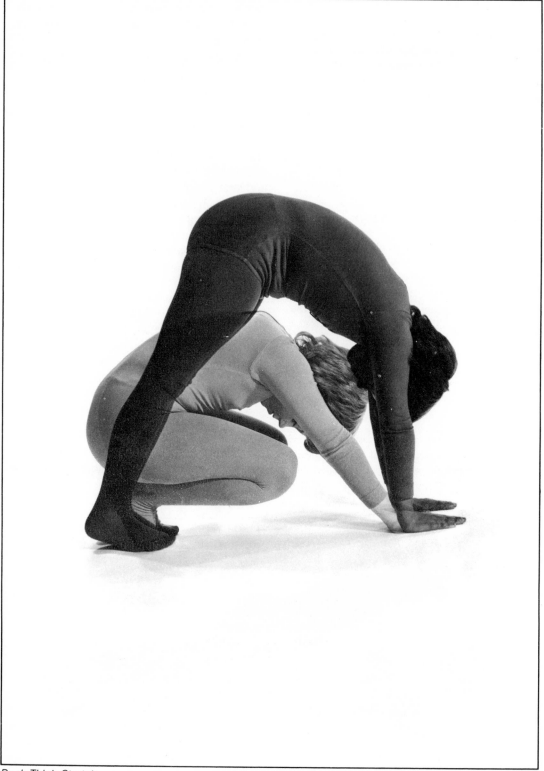

Back Thigh Stretch

6. PULL UP

Place a strong wood or metal pole across 2 chairs. Lie on back between chairs and grasp pole with hands about shoulder-width apart, palms facing the feet. When arms are fully extended the shoulders and head should remain on the floor. Keeping the body stiff, pull up until the chin is higher than the bar, supporting weight with the hands and heels. Then lower the body slowly to the floor. Note: A bar can easily be rigged up in a doorway. Those handy with tools can make a portable, adjustable bar. If the child is not strong enough to do a full pull up, 5 to 6 reps of the best pull up possible will soon develop enough strength to complete the movement.

Reps: 3x4 to 3x20   **Rest:** 15 sec.

Purpose: Develops strength and endurance in chest, shoulders, arms, upper back, and grip.

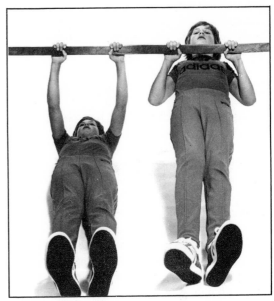

Pull Up

POSTURE

Studies in Canada and the United States have shown that no more than 20 per cent of children have what can be classed as good to fair posture. An equal number is in the very poor category. Children do not usually outgrow serious posture defects; they must be corrected. The longer they remain, the worse they get and the harder they are to put right.

Is good posture important?

If we build a bridge with a structural defect, it tends to collapse; so does the human body.

One of the most common defects, according to studies, is "kypho-lordosis" in which the upper back is rounded with the head slumped forward, while the lower back curves inward too far – the so-called "fatigue slump position". This is the position most of us assume when we lack energy and feel dejected.

It is interesting to note that this fault has a double-edged effect. Just as poor mental attitude can create poor posture, so poor posture can contribute to poor mental attitude.

7. BACK THIGH STRETCH

Crouch down with feet hip-width apart, knees and toes pointing straight ahead, hands flat on floor about 24 inches directly in front of the feet. Keeping hands on floor, slowly straighten legs until they are straight at the knees. Tuck the head into the knees. Hold for 3 seconds. Repeat 6 times, then move the hands 12 inches closer to the feet. Do another 6 reps. Then move hands right up to feet and try to do the exercise from this position.

At first it may be impossible to get the legs straight except from the first position. As flexibility develops, move hands in. Once the close-up position becomes easy, try the exercise with the backs of the hands on the floor.

Purpose: Develops flexibility in back thighs, and the lower back.

A posture defect invariably throws additional stress on some other parts of the body. Kypho-lordosis usually results in low-back problems later on in life; it also cramps the chest and the organs contained there, and causes fatigue and tension in the neck and upper back.

The fundamental cause of bad posture, apart from mental attitude, is lack of strength and flexibility. The individual tries to compensate for these shortcomings by using another muscle group not designed for the purpose, and the body slips out of alignment. When the body is erect and tall, the bone structure itself helps to bear most of the load; when it slumps forward, the muscles must do extra work. They become tense and tired.

Eighty-five per cent of all back problems result from lack of muscular strength, especially of the abdominal muscles. It is these muscles which hold the pelvic area in place; when they become weak, the pelvis slips and tilts forward throwing excessive stress onto the spinal column.

Posture defects caused by lack of strength and flexibility can be cured by special exercise. But there is another technique which is extremely useful with children: teach them to walk and sit tall. They will soon get the habit of holding their heads erect, chest high, and stomach in. It's a waste of time providing exercises if the youngster simply slips back into his or her usual slump once the workout is over.

Before launching your child on a fitness campaign, evaluate his or her posture so that you can include special exercises in the program for particular problems. While expert knowledge and techniques are required to provide a complete analysis, it is quite possible to detect the more common defects if you know what to look for.

Following is a list of some of the most common faults. Exercises which will help to repair them are listed on page 72, "What These Exercises Do". If you find that your child has unequal leg length or a low hip, consult your doctor for correctional procedures.

Common Posture Defects

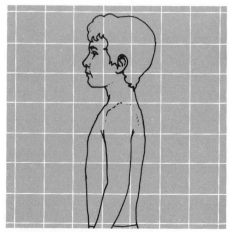

Correct Posture

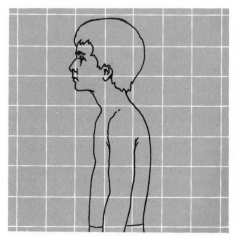

Forward Head   *Head tilted forward, with ear in front of shoulder line.*

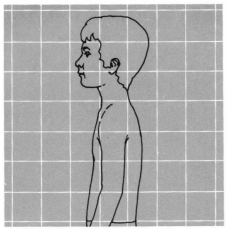

Shallow Chest *Absence of normal outward curve of chest beyond the shoulder line.*

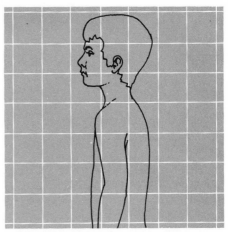

Round Shoulders *Shoulders in front of ear line and rounded upper back.*

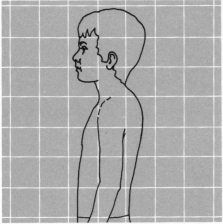

Kyphosis *Exaggerated outward curve of upper back.*

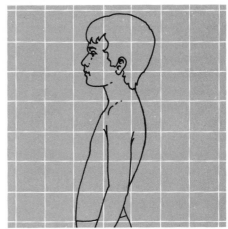

Lordosis *Exaggerated inward curve of lower back.*

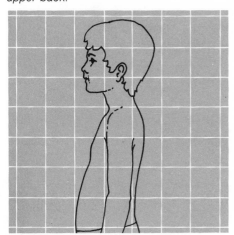

Protruding Abdomen *Lower abdomen extends forward beyond chest.*

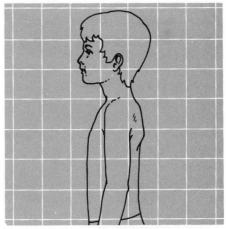

Protruding Scapulae *Shoulder blades not flat against back of chest.*

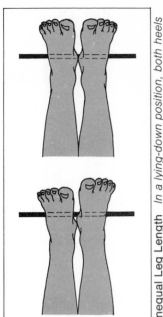

Unequal Leg Length *In a lying-down position, both heels do not touch the yardstick as they normally should. Note also that the ankle bones do not align.*

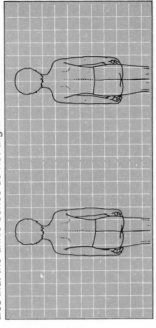

Low Hip *Top edge of one hip lower than the other.*

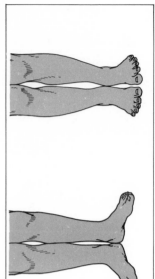

Charlie Chaplin Feet *Outward turn of feet results in structural stress throughout the body.*

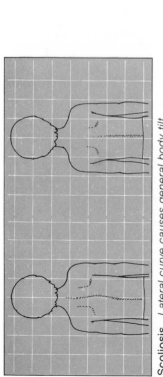

Scoliosis *Lateral curve causes general body tilt.*

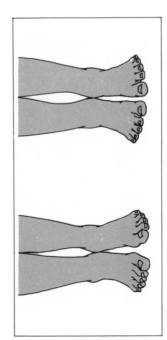

Bunched Toes *Inward angle of big and little toes.*

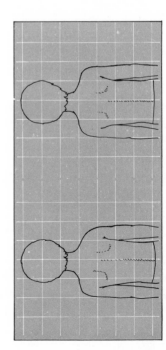

Dropped Shoulder *One shoulder below imaginary horizontal line.*

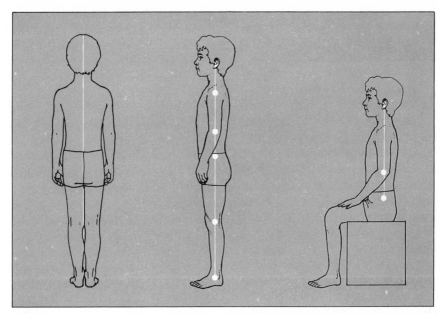

Correct Posture
This is your guide to correct posture. The vertical line indicates correct alignment of body parts. Seen from the back, it should extend through the exact center of the body, and the spine in particular should coincide with the plumb line. From the side, this plumb line should extend through the center of the head, ear, shoulder, hip and thigh, and pass just to the front of the ankle bone and through the middle of the arch of the foot. In correct sitting position, the feet are flat on the floor and parallel. The plumb line should pass through the center of the head, ear, shoulder, and hip joint.

FOR THE BUDDING ATHLETE

The program outlined earlier will take care of your child's minimum needs in such areas as strength, flexibility, and cardiovascular fitness. This does not mean that you should stop there. While 50 per cent may be considered a passing mark in school, the objective should still be excellence.

By achieving the highest possible level of physical fitness, your child can increase his or her capacity to excel. He will have more energy for both work and play and the ability to tolerate mental and physical stress, an ability which is one of the finest methods of health protection.

Your child may develop ambitions in sports, whether as a professional athlete or as an amateur. In this case, physical development becomes even more important. The requirements of excellence in contemporary sport are such that any physical weakness is soon exposed.

Perhaps you feel that you should not be concerned with "winning". But even a friendly game of tennis or non-competitive alpine skiing is more enjoyable when all the physical equipment is tuned up and available for use. The individual plays better and, equally important, recovers more quickly and is less prone to injury.

Following, then, is a review of some of the important factors of fitness which should receive special attention.

Strength

Not only is a weak child likely to be a weak adult, but the emotional and psychological handicaps imposed by muscular weakness have a profound effect on a child's development.

Additional strength can be developed

through proper training at any age, but attitudes toward physical exertion are conditioned by the successes we have when we are young. Strong children usually do better than weak ones in play, in sport, and in other areas where active physical participation is required.

Strength has a definite psychological and physiological advantage for the child. Many youngsters who want success and recognition in strenuous sports do not have the strength, coordination, and skill to match their enthusiasm and drive. This means they are prone to injury. Strength is one of the greatest protections any youngster can have against serious injury.

We are born with a body type which remains fairly constant throughout our life. Since the number of muscle fibers is fixed, some individuals can develop higher levels of strength than others. The tall, skinny youngster, for example, is not likely to become a world champion heavyweight weightlifter. He may, with hard training, become a top pole vaulter, however; and he or she can certainly do a great deal to develop the size and strength of the muscle fibers that are available.

The now-famous Kraus-Weber tests of North American children revealed some years ago that they rated much lower in muscular strength than did European children of the same age. This situation has not changed.

It has also been found that many school-age children suffer from posture problems which are not structural in origin, but simply the result of inadequate strength in the muscles responsible for holding the various parts of their bodies in alignment. The development of strength in these key muscles could eliminate many of the structural problems we suffer in later life, particularly kyphosis (hunchback) and many other spinal ailments.

A Basic Strength Program

Progressive weight training is the fastest and most effective way to develop muscular strength and size. By now the old myth about becoming muscle-bound has long been laid to rest: almost every major athlete in the world uses some form of resistance (weight) training in his or her development program. In progressive weight training the muscles are worked against gradually increased resistance, starting with light weights which can be easily handled. The muscles increase in strength as the weight increases, and/or develop added endurance, depending on the type of program being followed.

The advantage of weight training is that it can be started well within any individual's capabilities and is suitable for both boys and girls. It will give the child a solid foundation on which to build if he or she decides to develop the specific forms of strength required in gymnastics, shot putting, sprinting, pole vaulting, or downhill skiing.

This basic program is designed for boys and girls between the ages of 6 and 12. It requires a relatively inexpensive set of light weights: a barbell with collars to which weight discs can be added as required. If you like, you can improvise your own weights. However, children may be more highly motivated by equipment they associate with their athletic heroes.

Youngsters of 8 or younger may find the bar alone is sufficient for most of the exercises, at least to start. Even this may be too heavy for certain exercises such as the Pull Over. In this case, the *attempt* to do the drill is sufficient; combined with the other exercises, this will eventually develop sufficient strength so that the child can do the full drill properly.

Remember that it is always better to start with a weight that is a little too light than one that is too heavy. Start easily and progress gradually in simple stages.

This strength program should not be done every day. It is during the period of *recovery* from stress that the muscles are actually developing additional strength. Alternate strength work with the basic fitness program presented earlier in this chapter.

Progression

Start with just enough weight on the bar so the child can do 6 repetitions of each exercise without difficulty. They should be done in the order presented and with a short rest in between.

After every third workout or so, the child should try to add one repetition to each exercise. This progression should continue until 15 reps are being done. At this point, add 2 lbs. of weight and start again with 6 reps. Continue this progression.

After a good degree of strength has been developed, the work intensity can be boosted by doubling each exercise: 15 reps, rest, 15 more reps, rest; next exercise.

The first thing your youngster will probably want to do is test his or her strength with a maximum lift. This should not be permitted until the child has gained some experience in handling the weights and performing the exercises correctly. Once this stage has been reached, a strength test will add incentive and interest to the program. Keep records of performance and progress.

Always make sure the bar is evenly loaded and the collars are securely in place before starting any exercise. Weights can damage toes and floors if they fall off.

 PULL UP AND PRESS

Stand erect with feet comfortably apart. Hold barbell or weighted broomstick at arm's length across the thighs with slightly more than shoulder-width grip, with palms facing the thighs. Pull the bar straight up, keeping it close to the body. As it reaches shoulder height, lower the elbows and turn the hands so that they move under the bar ready for the press overhead. Now push the bar upwards until the arms are perfectly straight. Hold for a count of 3, then lower the bar slowly to the shoulders, rotate the hands over the top of the bar by lifting the elbows upward to the sides, and return it to the starting position. This completes one repetition. Breathe normally and do the exercise with a quick rhythm, making the arms and shoulders do the work. Do not sway the body.

> **Purpose:** Develops strength and endurance in the muscles of the arms, shoulders, and upper body.

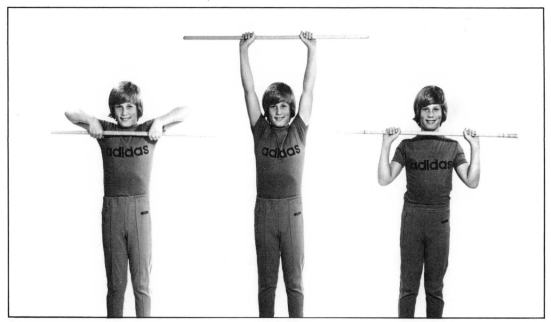

Pull Up and Press

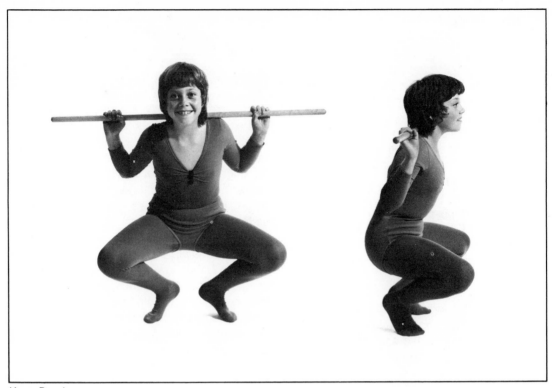

Knee Bend

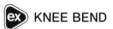 **KNEE BEND**

Stand erect with heels together and toes pointing outward at about 45 degrees. Hold a barbell or weighted broomstick across the shoulders behind the head. Breathe in deeply and do a half (not a full or deep) knee bend, allowing the heels to leave the floor. Return quickly to starting position, exhaling at the same time.

Keep the head and upper body as erect as possible throughout this exercise. The legs should do all the work. For variety, the feet may point straight ahead, be widely spaced, or kept flat on the floor during the squat.

> **Purpose:** Develops strength and endurance in leg muscles.

 PULL OVER

Lie on back with barbell or weighted broomstick at arm's length above the chest, hands about shoulder-width apart, palms facing toward feet. Breathe in and lower the barbell slowly past the head to the floor, keeping the arms straight and reaching as far back as possible. Hold full stretch for a count of 3, then while exhaling, pull the bar slowly back to starting position.

It is important to inhale and exhale deeply when doing this exercise, and to keep the arms absolutely straight. The benefits can be increased once a certain amount of strength has been developed by doing the exercise while lying on a bench, or with a pillow under the upper back to increase the range of movement.

> **Purpose:** Develops flexibility and strength of the muscles of the rib cage and shoulders.

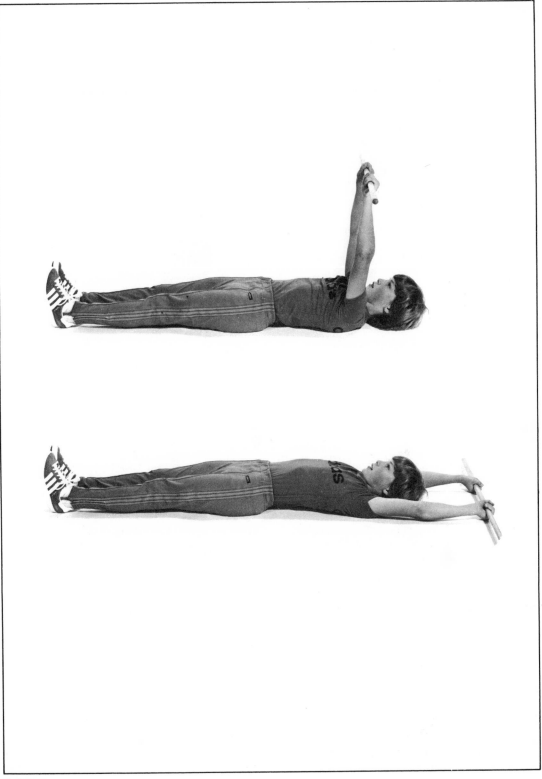

Pull Over

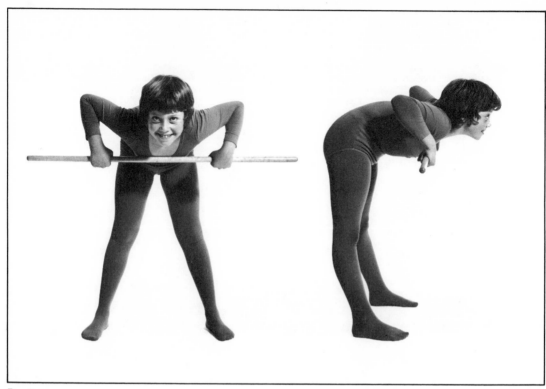

Rowing

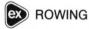 ROWING

Stand with feet about shoulder-width apart, upper body bent forward so back is parallel to floor. Hold barbell at full arm's length, hands slightly more than shoulder-width apart, palms facing feet. The knees may be slightly bent if this feels more comfortable. Exhale and pull the bar straight up, bending the elbows out to the sides, until it touches chest. Hold for count of 3, then lower bar to starting position, inhaling at the same time.

Keep the back parallel to the floor at all times so the muscles of the arms, shoulders, and upper back have to do the work. For variety use a narrower grip from time to time, and pull the bar up to the waist instead of the chest.

Purpose: Develops strength and endurance in the muscles of the upper back, shoulders and arms.

CURL

Stand erect with feet about shoulder-width apart and barbell or weighted broomstick held at full arm's length across the thighs. Grip the barbell at slightly more than shoulder width with the palms facing away from the legs. Raise bar to shoulder height by bending elbows, keeping the upper arms in place (the elbows should not move back behind the body). Make the biceps do the work. Lower the bar *steadily* to the starting position (Do not drop it – the biceps should continue to work during this movement). Only the forearms move in this exercise, the upper body should not swing back and forth, and the upper arms must remain at the sides.

Purpose: Develops strength and endurance in the arms and hands.

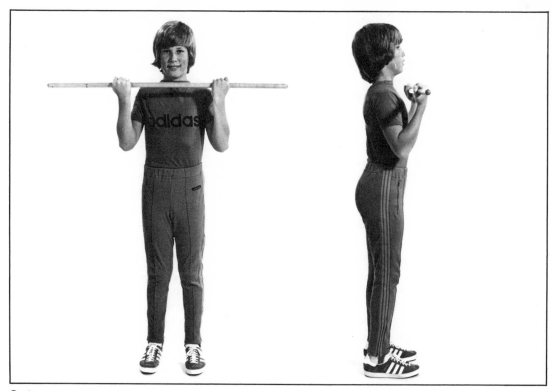

Curl

Endurance

The child with low endurance who gets winded quickly and lacks energy is a prime candidate for a medical examination. If no health problem is evident, the best answer is endurance training.

The basic exercise program presented earlier in this chapter is an excellent starting point. But running is probably the best single developer of heart-respiratory endurance for the young person, and will build good basic stamina. Your youngster should be encouraged to run as much as possible and to play games involving the leg muscles: soccer, lacrosse, tennis, basketball, swimming, track and field. Baseball and softball are not as effective since the bursts of activity are few and lacking in intensity. Moreover, there is mounting evidence that hard throwing at an early age can damage the joints and sockets of growing bones.

Similarly the body contact of football or hockey may be damaging for young children.

Some parents worry that their children are overdoing things when they come home exhausted at the end of a hard day. Relax: It's very hard for a strong, healthy, well-fed 8-year-old to exceed the recuperative capacities of his or her growing body. But do make sure that their basic diet is sound (see the section on feeding your athletic son and daughter in Chapter 7) and pay special attention to replenishing vital nutrients after hard activity.

The Russians start training their potential marathon champions at the age of 8! This doesn't mean that you have to send your young athlete out on a 26-mile run, but if your child shows aptitude and inclination, track clubs offer an ideal source of endurance training. Ascertain if your local club offers instruction in your child's age group. Starting your youngster with others who are more mature and stronger may be discouraging, and he or she could lose interest. In this case you can probably do a better job of coaching yourself. Get a good book on the subject, and read up on the principles of interval training and progression to ensure that everyone gets maximum benefit from effort.

Canadian cardiac specialist Dr. Gordon Cumming was asked about possible injury to the heart of a young athlete who undertakes hard training. His answer was:

"I have been doing pediatric cardiology for 16 years and I have never seen such a heart strain. The heart enlarges through training – as much as 25 per cent – but this is fine; it has not been proven to be harmful. But when you see a large heart not associated with training and the capacity to exercise is not correspondingly increased, then that is a different story. Give young athletes a thorough medical first and then let them go, and stop worrying."[3]

Flexibility

Children are born flexible. The aging process seems to be one of progressive loss of free movement until rigor mortis sets in. Sedentary living hastens the process; the more we sit, the faster the muscles and joints lose their ability for a full range of movement. Children who watch a lot of television are particularly susceptible to this problem.

Does it matter if your child can't touch his toes? The answer is yes. In sport, flexibility provides protection from injuries such as muscle tears, and contributes to skill, agility, and endurance. It assists in developing and sustaining good posture since correct body positions come easily and naturally. The flexible person will have much greater freedom of movement, less physical discomfort, less muscular tension, and increased freedom from injury for the rest of his life. He will stay physically younger, longer.

The following exercises are designed to create flexibility in the most important muscle groups and joints. Your child need not do all of them. Any exercise which he or she finds particularly difficult should be added to the basic fitness program outlined earlier. Those which are easy can be ignored, since ease of movement indicates adequate flexibility in that particular area.

However, people change. It would be wise to refer to these exercises every six months or so to see if any of them are starting to become difficult to perform. These can then be done for a few weeks to nip the problem in the bud.

These exercises are also excellent warm-up drills before games and practices, and can help the individual recover quickly from hard effort by loosening up muscles which may have become tight through exertion and the accumulation of fatigue products such as lactic acid.

All stretching exercises should be done *slowly*. Quick, bouncy movements are not as effective and may be stressful.

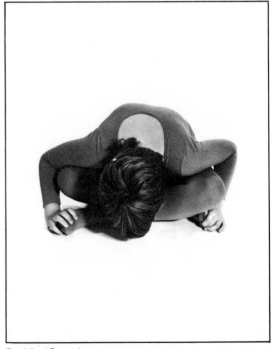

Buddha Stretch

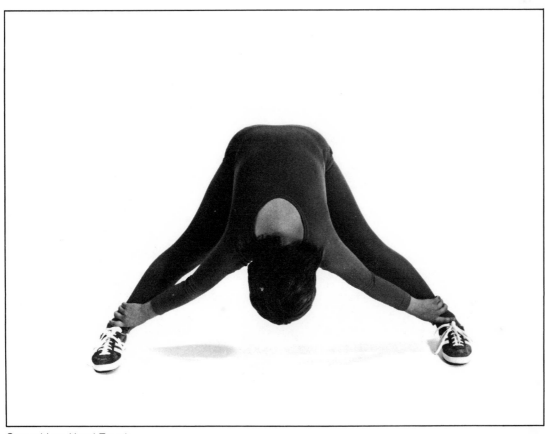

Spread Leg Head Touch

 BUDDHA STRETCH

Sit cross-legged with each hand clasped across the opposite foot (right hand over left, left hand over right). Pull down slowly, trying to touch head to floor between knees. Hold for 3 seconds, then relax and return to starting position. Parent can press down gently on back to help out at first.

Reps: 6 to 12.

Purpose: Develops flexibility in knees, hip, back, and shoulder areas.

 SPREAD LEG HEAD TOUCH

Stand with feet spread wider than shoulder-width apart, toes pointing forward. Reach down and, keeping knees absolutely straight, clasp the ankles or as close to the ankles as you can reach. Pull down *slowly* and try to touch head to floor. Hold maximum stretch for a count of 3 and return to starting position.

Initially, there may be difficulty with this drill. It is permissable for the parent to press down *gently* on the upper back to assist the child in getting his or her head to the floor. The knees must not be bent.

Reps: 6 to 12.

Purpose: Develops flexibility in low back and back thighs.

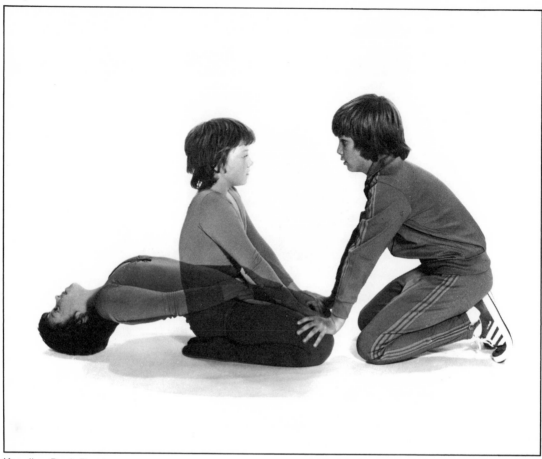

Kneeling Back Bend

 KNEELING BACK BEND

Kneel on floor with knees about 6 inches apart, toes pointing straight back. Hands should be palm down on the front thighs. Bend backward, trying to touch top of head to floor. Hold for a count of 3 and return to the starting position. The parent may have to hold down the knees during the first few days. Emphasize the arching or bowing of the back as the child leans back to increase the flexibility load on the chest.

Reps: 6 to 12.

Purpose: Develops flexibility in chest, front thighs, and abdomen.

 LEG CIRCLING

Lie on back and raise right leg with knee straight and locked until it is pointing straight up in the air. Move it in as wide a circle as possible, first one direction, then the other, keeping knees straight. Continue for 15 seconds, lower leg to floor, and repeat with left leg.

Reps: 30 sec. to 90 sec.

Purpose: Develops flexibility in the hip area.

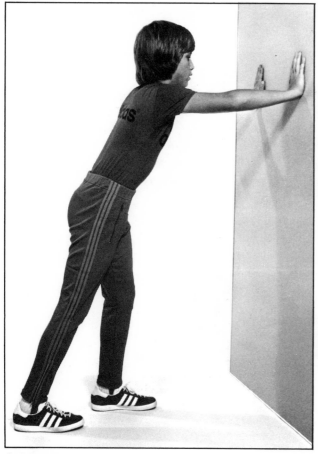

Calf Stretch

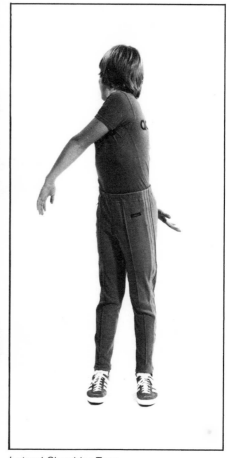

Lateral Shoulder Turn

 CALF STRETCH

Stand with hands on wall about 12 inches apart, feet close together. Keeping heels flat on floor, slowly shuffle feet back until they are as far away from wall as possible. Slowly lift heels and then lower them to the floor again, each time trying to move them back a little more.

Reps: 10 to 20.

Purpose: Develops flexibility in calf muscles.

 LATERAL SHOULDER TURN

Stand comfortably with feet about 6 inches apart, stomach in, chest high, head erect, arms hanging at sides. Swing shoulders as far around to the left as possible, the objective being to turn the upper body completely around. Hold maximum stretch for 3 seconds, then swing shoulders around to the opposite side as far as possible.

The head and arms are allowed to swing freely around in conjunction with shoulders. Care should be taken that the level of the shoulders remains constant during the turn.

Reps: 6 to 12.

Purpose: Develops flexibility of back, mid-section and upper body.

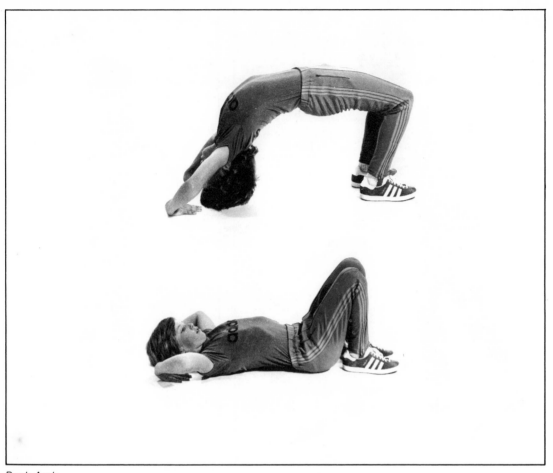

Back Arch

 BACK ARCH

Lie on back with legs well bent and feet on floor directly under knees. Place hands on floor overhead, fingers pointing toward feet. Raise body as high as possible, forming an arch. (Parent may have to provide assistance at first.) Try to move hands and feet closer together to increase height of arch. Hold maximum stretch for count of 5, return to starting position.

Reps: 6 to 8.

Purpose: Develops hip, chest, shoulder, and arm flexibility. Will also develop some arm, shoulder, and back strength.

Agility

If your child tends to be awkward, there are many good remedies: gymnastics, ballet or other dancing classes, figure skating or power skating (many figure-skating clubs now teach power skating for hockey), handball, volleyball, badminton, squash, and skiing. A year or two in a good gymnastics program is hard to beat for developing all-round agility and coordination.

Studies have shown that a majority of children who are hurt in sports and in accidents have low levels of agility. Agility training will not only help children in their sports activities, but will improve their safety and give them confidence and poise.

Relaxation

We think of tension as primarily an adult problem, but it also affects children. This is particularly true now that television has replaced physical activity as a principal source of entertainment – nervous and emotional stimulation has increased, but the means of releasing the resulting tensions has decreased.

When the child lacks physical outlets, tension may manifest itself in many ways: excessive nervousness about exams and other school crises, irritability, mischievousness, inability to concentrate, nervous stomach, emotional outbursts.

Reports from Sweden indicate that children who had been taught the art of relaxation learned faster, retained their knowledge longer, and were generally healthier and more stable emotionally.

The child who has learned to control his muscles so that he or she can relax them at will has a skill that will be invaluable throughout life. Chapter 8, "How to Reduce Tension and Learn to Relax", describes how this skill can be developed.

Nutrition and Weight Control

It's hard to overvalue the role of nutrition in developing fitness and health – it's probably the single most important factor. Yet surveys have shown imbalances and deficiencies in what young people eat. Many eat too much, particularly junk foods, and are overweight. Nutrition Canada studies show that 20 to 30 per cent of children lack sufficient calcium for healthy bone and teeth formation; a similar percentage lack adequate Vitamin D which aids in the absorption of bone-building minerals; three quarters of all adolescent girls studied were short of iron and were developing anemia. These are just a few examples. The shortfall of vital food elements in the average diet is amazing.

Children who are overweight and undernourished lack speed, agility, energy, and endurance, apart from the obvious health hazard created by the absence of essential proteins, vitamins, and minerals. Heightened anxiety and nervousness often result.

This is the era of easily accessible junk foods, usually dispensed by machines. Even some schools offer this type of diet in their cafeterias. It's easy for parents to fall into the habit of relying on such time-and-effort savers as a major food source for their children, who learn to prefer them to more wholesome foods. The quickie pre-packaged complete meals are almost as bad, because much of the nutritional value is steamed and cooked out of the food during the packaging.

One of the most important steps in any fitness campaign is to make sure the diet is not just adequate, but excellent. Chapter 7, "Nutrition" explains the daily needs of growing children and provides guidelines which can help you safeguard your youngsters' future.

Notes

Chapter 1

[1]LAURENCE E. MOREHOUSE AND LEONARD GROSS, *Total Fitness* (New York: Simon and Schuster, 1975), p. 75.

[2]EDWARD STIEGLITZ, *Living Through the Older Years* (Ann Arbor: University of Michigan Press, 1949).

[3]HELEN B. PRYOR, ''Posture'', in the *Encyclopedia of Sport Sciences and Medicine* (Toronto: Collier-Macmillan, 1971), p. 3.

[4]KATHARINE F. WELLS, *Posture Exercise Handbook: A Progressive Sequence Approach*. Copyright © 1963 The Ronald Press Company, New York. (pp. 3 and 4)

[5]HERBERT DEVRIES, in *Proceedings of the International Symposium on the Art and Science of Coaching* (October 1974), pp. 315 and 316.

[6]From *Stress Without Distress* by HANS SELYE, M.D. Copyright © 1974 by Hans Selye, M.D. Reprinted by permission of J. B. Lippincott Company and of the Canadian Publishers, McClelland and Stewart Limited, Toronto. (p. 27)

Chapter 2

[1]PER-OLOF ASTRAND, *Textbook of Work Physiology* (New York: McGraw-Hill, 1970), p. 93.

[2]Copyright © 1975 by SHIRLEY MOTTER LINDE AND FRANK A. FINNERTY, JR., M.D. From the book *High Blood Pressure*, published by David McKay Co., Inc. Reprinted by permission of the publisher. (p. 93)

[3]JEAN MAYER, *Overweight: Causes, Cost, and Control* (Englewood Cliffs, N.J.: Prentice-Hall, Inc., 1968).

[4]RICHARD B. STUART AND BARBARA DAVIS, *Slim Chance in a Fat World* (Champaign, Ill.: Research Press, 1972).

[5]LLOYD PERCIVAL in *Canadian Family Physician* (July 1972).

Chapter 4

[1]GEORGE F. BRADY, ''Muscular Endurance'', in *Enclopedia of Sport Sciences and Medicine*, p. 288.

Chapter 5

[1]D. SINCLAIR, ''Stitches'', in *Encyclopedia of Sport Sciences and Medicine*, pp. 260-61.

[2]LINDSAY A. BELCH, ''Exercise and Pregnancy'', *Sports and Fitness Instructor* (March 1973).

Chapter 6

[1]IRWIN ROSS in *Sports and Fitness Instructor* (March 1973).

Chapter 7

[1]L. JEAN BOGERT, GEORGE M. BRIGGS, AND DORIS CALLOWAY, *Nutrition and Physical Fitness* (Philadelphia: W. B. Saunders, 1973).

[2]L. PROKOP, ''Vitamin Supplementation'', in *Encyclopedia of Sport Sciences and Medicine*, p. 128.

[3]ELIZABETH CHANT ROBERTSON AND MARGARET I. WOOD, *Today's Child*, 1971. Reprint by permission of Pagurian Press Limited. © Pagurian Press Limited.

[4]*Overweight: Causes, Cost, and Control.*

Chapter 8

[1]*Stress Without Distress*, p. 47.

[2]*Stress Without Distress*, p. 130.

Chapter 9

[1]WILHELM RAAB AND HANS KRAUS, *Hypokinetic Disease*, 1971. Courtesy of Charles C Thomas, Publisher, Springfield, Illinois.

Chapter 10

[1]ELAINE TANNER in *Proceedings of the International Symposium on the Art and Science of Coaching*.

[2]GORDON CUMMING in *Proceedings*.

Metric Conversion Table

Length	1 inch = **25.4** mm 1 foot = **30.48** cm 1 yard = **0.9144** m 1 mile = **1.609 344** km	Force	1 pound-force = 4.448 222 N 1 kilogram-force = **9.806 65** N
Area	1 square inch = **6.4516** cm² 1 square foot = **9.290 304** dm² 1 square yard = **0.836 127 4** m² 1 acre = 0.404 685 6 ha 1 square mile = 2.589 988 km²	Pressure	1 pound-force per square inch (psi) = 6.894 757 kPa 1 inch of mercury (0°C) = 3.386 39 kPa 1 mm of mercury (0°C) = 133.322 Pa 1 standard atmosphere (atm) = **101.325** kPa
Volume	1 cubic inch = **16.387 064** cm³ 1 cubic foot = 28.316 85 dm³ (or litres) 1 cubic yard = 0.764 555 m³ 1 fluid ounce = 28.413 062 cm³ 1 gallon = **4.546 090** dm³ (or litres)	Energy, Work	1 British thermal unit (Btu) = 1055.06 J 1 foot pound force = 1.355 818 J 1 calorie (international) = **4.1868** J 1 kilowatt hour (kW h) = **3.6** MJ
Mass	1 ounce (avoirdupois) = 28.349 523 g 1 pound (avoirdupois) = **0.453 592 37** kg 1 ton (short, 2000 lb) = **907.184 74** kg	Power	1 horsepower (550 ft.lbf/s) = 745.6999 W 1 horsepower (electric) = **746** W
Temperature	(5/9) x (number of degrees Fahrenheit **−32** = number of degrees Celsius		
Speed	1 mile per hour = **0.447 04** m/s = **1.609 344** km/h		

Source: *The Metric Guide* by the Council of Ministers of Education, Canada

factors which are exact are in bold type

Index